DIABETIC
AIR FRYER COOKBOOK :

All The Secrets To Prepare the tastiest dishes with the Air Fryer. 250 Quick and Easy Recipes that Prevent Diabetes and Also Make You Lose Weight.

AUTHOR: CHERYL SHEA

Table of Contents

Introduction

Air frying is actually a very new cooking concept and wasn't introduced to the market until 2010. Prior to this, the only way to fry was to submerge food in a vat of cooking oil. This new technology, however, finally allowed home cooks to get the same results that restaurants achieve, but without the use of cumbersome deep fryers and huge quantities of oil. The result is a way to get perfectly crispy fried foods without the mess of deep frying, and using only a tiny amount of oil. Not only is air frying easier, it's also much healthier!

The health benefits of air frying are perhaps the best reason to consider this cooking method. The main problem with traditional deep frying isn't the food you are cooking, but rather the oil used in the cooking process. Traditional deep frying requires you to fully submerge your food in oil, and as a result, your food absorbs a lot of that oil. The problem is that oil contains a lot of calories, fat, and often cholesterol. Because these oils mix with the carbohydrates in your food, you end up with one of the unhealthiest combinations possible. Air fryers, on the other hand, only use a tiny amount of oil. Because they are able to use circulating hot air to cook your food, the amount of oil can be greatly reduced, which means you are not eating nearly as much fat. This leads to lighter foods which are not only better for you, they actually taste lighter and are more flavorful.

Aside from the calorie count, the biggest negative factor of oil frying is that it is downright dangerous. How many times have you thrown something into oil and then ran the other direction to avoid the hot oil splatter? It's not only unpleasant, it's unsafe.

If there is one concern more important than burning your skin it may be burning your whole house down. The lack of oil frying means there is no oil to start a kitchen fire which could eventually lead to a house fire.

Chapter 1. How The Air Fryer Works

Air Fryer is a kitchen appliance with versatility and ingenious design, with patented technology that cooks food by super- heated air. It heats up within a minute, and there is a swift flow of hot air within the dedicated chamber making food to cook evenly while using less oil.

This game-changing kitchen appliance has the rapid air circulation technology which enables hot air to surround the food you want to cook at high speeds to develop the crispy food we all crave for. On top of the delicious crunchy food, little oil is used in the process which makes it a guilt-free delicacy!

Tips to Prepare Healthy Foods in Air Fryer

1. Vegetables are one of the easiest foods to cook in Air Fryer. A wide variety of plants can be cooked, be it delicate beans to root vegetables. For the best cooking experience, firstly, soak the vegetables, especially the harder ones, in cold water for 15 - 20 minutes. Then after, dry them using a clean kitchen towel.

2. Roasting with air is a new cooking trend you have to try because you can finally prepare your winter favorites

3. Flip foods when half the cooking time is attained; Just as you would if you were cooking on a grill or in a skillet, you need to turn foods over so that they brown evenly.

4. You can bake your favorite recipes in your Air Fryer but always check with the machine's manual before using new baking ware with Air Fryer

5. Aim at cooking your food to the desired doneness because the recipes are flexible and they are designed for all Air Fryer models.

If you feel that the food needs more cooking time, then adjust it and cook for a few more minutes. It is not necessary to stick to a recipe time, as certain ingredients can vary in their size and firmness from one place to another

6. When it comes to cooking time, it changes depending on the particular Air Fryer model, the size of food, food pre-preparation and so on.

For shorter cooking cycles, you should preheat Air Fryer for about 3 - 4 minutes. otherwise, if you put the ingredients into the cold cooking basket, the cooking time needs to be increased to 3 additional minutes.

7. Use a good quality oil spray to brush food and cooking basket; it is also helpful for easy cleanup

How Does An Air Fryer Differ From A Convection Oven Or A Turbocharger?

While there's not much difference between the air fryer, turbocharger, and convection oven, there is enough difference to make it worth investigating to find the perfect fit for your personal needs.

Much like the air fryer, a convection oven circulates superheated air around the food, but there are very few portable/smaller-sized convection ovens, and usually, only the most expensive ones have a fan that circulates the air more evenly.

A turbo grill works using infrared/halogen light heat. As a radiant heat, it travels through the pot, and vice only rises as it does in a convection oven.

The air fryer uses an ingenious combination of both methods, differing from the convection oven because heat circulates everywhere (vice rising to the top) through the fan, and not through the turbo because there is typically no heating element in the top of a fryer from where the heat comes out. They use electrical energy to create their heat; a lot of power!

Characteristics of Air Fryers

Air Fryers in the market today vary in many of the features they offer. In general terms, halogen oven opinions fryers have the same right to fame: to provide consumers with the same flavor and texture of traditionally "fried" foods, but by using a fraction of the oil used by traditional fryers.

This characteristic not only makes them healthier for the heart, but also prevents many of the burns that can occur when it comes to getting the perfect fried foods.

Most air fryers offer a variety of cooking methods, and some have pre-programmed settings for cooking different types of food. You can cook so many things in an air fryer, including but not limited to meat, shrimp, chicken, and cakes.

What about pastries?

Yes! An advantage of the air fryer being similar in concept to a convection oven is to be able to 'bake' in an air fryer, but without needing the time[AT1], you would typically need to use a regular oven.

However, baking in an air fryer often requires a separate baking sheet, and currently, there are only two on the market that offer this accessory.

Some air fryers also promote their near-endless cooking functionalities by offering a reasonably cavernous kitchen space in comparison to their competing air fryers.

Why should you have one?

Why? The list is endless! There are some quite surprising reasons to have an air fryer in today's day and age. Although they try to isolate themselves as "oil-free" fryers, most air fryers have a lot of versatility in what they can be used for. They also offer quick and easy options for today's busy family looking to cook healthier meals.

air fryers also offer a reheating option that most broilers do not have, and air fryers are not as bulky as most other convection ovens.

The growing concerns about electromagnetic radiation in microwave ovens are sending more and more consumers looking for better ways to cook meals quickly, and an air fryer meets that demand.

The industry leader, Philips, manufactures different lines of air fryers. They are the best at the price level. While the cost of a good Philips air fryer might cause a consumer to hesitate, most of the customers swear they would not buy anything else.

Another thing to take into consideration is capacity. If you are looking to feed a family of four or more people, you must invest in an air fryer that has the functionality to cook more food at once.

Most air fryers are ideal for one or two people, possibly three. However, many of them are not necessarily the perfect appliance for large family dishes.

How Does Air Fryer Toaster Oven Works?

The technology of the Air Fryer Toaster Oven is very simple. Fried foods get their crunchy texture because hot oil heats foods quickly and evenly on their surface. Oil is an excellent heat conductor, which helps with fast and simultaneous cooking across all of the ingredients. For decades cooks have used convection ovens to try to mimic the effects of frying or cooking the whole surface of the food. But the air never circulates quickly enough to achieve that delicious surface crisp we all love in fried foods.

With this mechanism, the air is circulated on high degrees, up to 200° C, to "air fry" any food such as fish, chicken or chips, etc. This technology has changed the whole idea of cooking by reducing the fat up to 80% compared to old-fashioned deep fat frying.

The Air Fryer Toaster Oven cooking releases the heat through a heating element which cooks the food in a healthier and more appropriate way. There's also an exhaust fan right above the cooking chamber which provides the food required airflow. This way food is cooked with constant heated air. This leads to the same heating temperature reaching every single part of the food that is being cooked. So, this is only grill and the exhaust fan that is helping the Air Fryer Toaster Oven to boost air at a constantly high speed in order to cook healthy food with less fat.

The internal pressure increases the temperature that will then be controlled by the exhaust system. Exhaust fan also releases filtered extra air to cook the food in a much healthier way. Air Fryer Toaster Oven has no odor at all and it is absolutely harmless making it user and environment-friendly.

The Simplicity of Air Fryer Cooking

As you may know, the air fryer has become a sort of craze these last few years, and there are many reasons why. First off, it is extremely easy to use that even kids can run the machine. Therefore, even if you are not a master chef, you will be able to fry delicious and nutritious meals for you and your family.

Another reason why people love the air fryer so much is that it uses very little oil.

This helps to maintain the fried foods in your healthy diet since you will not be consuming the greasy fat that you normally would. In addition, it is quicker most of the time!

Many of the models come with a menu specific to what item you are cooking such as French fries, cakes, and fish. There also is the ease of pressing the settings you require and letting the air fryer work its magic while you do other tasks. It really cannot get much easier when everything is already figured out for you.

The cleanup is a breeze when it comes to air frying. Because there is no oil, you will not have to scrub pots and pans every night. There are also removable parts that you can easily stack in the dishwasher.

The beauty of the fryer is that you can insert oven-safe baking pans, ramekins, and silicone bakeware inside the basket with no issue. This results to less cleanup since you will be serving from the dish you are using to bake.

The time factor also helps make the air fryer very simple to use. You will find that most of your favorite dishes will now be served even more quickly and taste just as delicious.

This is especially the case with your fried foods, as you will still have the fantastic crunch factor that we all crave with deep-fried foods. Besides, since you are using little oil, you will be consuming much fewer calories while still enjoying your meal to the fullest.

If you find this cookbook So, are you ready to get started with these exciting recipes? Let us get to the good stuff: the recipes. Enjoy!

Chapter 2. Advice On Which Accessories To Use For Cooking Delicious Recipes.

Function Keys

- **Button / Play/Pause Button**

This Play/Pause button allows you to pause during the middle of the cooking so you can shake the air fryer basket or flip the food to ensure it cooks evenly.

- **-/+ Button /Minus/Plus Button**

This button is used to change the time or temperature.

- **Keep Warm**

This function keeps your food warm for 30 minutes.

- **Food Presets**

This button gives you the ability to cook food without second-guessing. The time and temperature are already set, so new users find this setting useful.

- **Roast or Broil**

You can roast or broil with this setting. When using a conventional oven, you need to brown the meat before roasting. You can skip this step when cooking with an air fryer.

- **Dehydrate**

This setting cooks and dries food at a low temperature for a few hours. With this option, you can create your own beef jerky or dried fruit.

Features of Your Air Fryer

1. Portable: The cooking device is portable. The air fryer is designed to be easily transferred from your kitchen storage cabinet to the countertop or elsewhere

2. Automatic temperature control: You get perfectly cooked food every time with an air fryer.

3. Digital touch screen: You don't have to learn complicated cooking skills, simplicity is inbuilt with an air fryer. With a few taps on the touch panel's screen, you can cook a variety of foods.

4. Timer and buzzer: No need to worry about overcooking your food. The timer and buzzer will let you know when your food is cooked.

Advice on Using the Air Fryer

1. Firstly, you are able to set the temperature based on the thing you need and allow it to preheat for just a few minutes before you decide to place the food in.

2. Then open it up and put the meals within the air fryer. Close it and allow the food to prepare based on the timing you've set. It will not take enough time regardless of what you're cooking.

3. You may use a little bit of cooking spray or splash some oil around the food before putting it in. This can help to prevent the meals from getting stuck towards the pan. The oil likewise helps to create food a bit crispier and provides the taste of standard fried food.

4. Halfway with the set time or perhaps in between times, provide the air fryer just a little shake so the air inside circulates easily and your meals are completely cooked.

5. Other than frying, you can test other cooking methods while using additional parts the air flyers usually include. You should use the grill or baking tray in compliance using the instructions that include the environment fryer.

6. Another factor to bear in mind is you shouldn't overcrowd the fryer by putting an excessive amount of food inside it. Put small batches of food within the air fryer to ensure that there's enough room for this all to maneuver and prepare evenly. Overcrowding won't let it move and a few parts is going to be left uncooked. The cooking can also be elevated if you devote an excessive amount of at the same time.

7. In the situation of marinated food, allow it to be as dry as you possibly can before placing it within the air fryer. Wet food may cause splattering in addition to an excessive amount of smoke being released in the fryer.

8. The separator that will get the environment fryer can be put among layers of food in order to prepare various things concurrently. Just make certain the temperature needed is identical for those products or they will not be cooked evenly.

9. Pre-packaged meals may also be made while using air fryer. Lower the suggested oven temperature and hang the environment fryer after your meals are placed within it. Additionally, it cuts down on the normal cooking considerably.

10. For baking food, you should use the baking pan provided or purchase one individually. You do not need a stove to bake some muffins any longer and also you have them cooked even faster than in the past.

11. Roasting meals are also simpler than using conventional methods. It doesn't take considerable time but you just get individuals healthy and attractive roasted veggies or meats that you simply love. For grilling food, put the grill layer inside as well as your food on the top from it. You don't need to help keep flipping the meals over as with a conventional grill.

This will make things much easier. Give it a shake following a couple of moments for much better air flow.

As possible clearly see in the information above, significantly less efforts are needed while the food is cooking. Make use of the simple mechanism and prepare a number of different meals every single day.

Air Fryer vs. Deep Fryer

1. Oil usage: Air fryers use less oil, this means using an air fryer costs you less. You need to use a lot more oil when deep-frying. Although you can reuse the oil, most health experts do not recommend it.

2. Healthy cooking: Fried foods such as air fried French fries contain up to 80% less fat in comparison to deep-fried French fries.

3. Cleaning: Compared to a deep fryer, cleaning an air fryer is easy. You need to clean the deep fryer and the oil vapor that settles on the kitchen walls and countertop.

4. Safety: An air fryer is safe to use. With a deep fryer, there is always a risk of accidents.

5. Multiple uses: You can only fry in a deep-fryer. On the other hand, you can cook in many different ways in an air fryer.

- Healthier, oil-free meals

- It eliminates cooking odors through internal air filters

- Makes cleaning easier due to lack of oil grease

- Air Fryer Toaster Oven is able to bake, grill, roast and fry providing more options

- A safer method of cooking compared to deep frying with exposed hot oil

- Has the ability to set and leave as most models and it includes a digital timer

The Air Fryer Toaster Oven is an all-in-one that allows cooking to be easy and quick. It also leads to a lot of possibilities once you get to know it. Once you learn the basics and become familiar with your Air Fryer Toaster Oven, you can feel free to experiment and modify the recipes in the way you prefer. You can prepare a wide number of dishes in the Air Fryer Toaster Oven and you can adapt your favorite stove-top dish so it becomes Air Fryer Toaster Oven–friendly. It all boils down to variety and lots of options, right?

Air Fryer vs. Convection Oven

1. Less hazardous: An air fryer gives you a one-stop cooking solution. With ovens, you often must cook food in a pan for a few minutes to bring out the color and aromas before putting it in the oven.

2. Safe: You can open and close the air fryer without the risk of burning yourself. A traditional oven presents a risk of fire.

3. Time: You can cook faster in an air fryer.

4. Cleaning: Cleaning your air fryer is easy. On the other hand, cleaning an oven is time-consuming.

Tips for the Perfect Air Fry

1. Find a place in your kitchen where it will always be easy to access the air fryer, to the point that you simply need to open the cooking container and add your ingredients.

2. Different recipes require different temperatures to ensure that the food is cooked properly. Follow the recipe as precisely as possible to ensure that your food tastes delicious.

3. Aluminum foil helps with cleaning and is often used to add even more gradual control to the cooking process for the ingredients.

4. Add a dash of water when cooking fatty foods. You will notice a small drawer at the bottom of your air fryer. This is where you can add a splash of water when you are cooking foods that are high in fat. If the fat becomes too hot and drips to the bottom for too long, it can sometimes start to smoke. Adding vegetables prevents smoke. But if you are only cooking meat, then it is a good idea to add water to prevent the unpleasant smoke from rising.

5. Do not overcrowd the air fryer's cooking basket with too many ingredients. Make sure that the ingredients are all at one level, especially if you are preparing meat.

6. Flip foods halfway through the cooking time if you want both sides of your food to have a crispy coating.

7. Do not worry about opening the air fryer mid-cycle. Unlike other cooking methods, the air fryer doesn't lose heat intensity if you open it in the middle of cooking. Once you close the top again, the device will go back to cooking temperature and continue to cook the food.

8. There is a basket at the bottom of the air fryer to collect grease. If you take out both the cooking basket and the bottom basket at the same time and you tip them over, the grease from the bottom will be transferred onto your plate along with food. So, remove the bottom basket before serving the food.

9. Clean the air fryer after every use. Leftover food particles can turn into mold, develop bacteria, and cause unpleasant after-effects. To avoid this, clean the air fryer after every use.

10. Once you clean the air fryer, assemble everything. The air fryer will dry itself within a few minutes.

Here Are Some Of The Cooking Techniques That You Can Use With This Appliance:

- Fry: You can avoid oil when cooking, but a small amount adds crunch and flavor to your food.

- Roast: You can produce high quality roasted food in the air fryer

- Bake: You can bake bread, cookies, and pastries.

- Grill: You can effectively grill your food, no mess.

To start cooking, you just need to spray the fryer basket with some cooking spray or put in a little cooking oil, add the ingredients, and adjust the temperature and time.

Troubleshooting

1. Food not cooking perfectly: Follow the recipe exactly. Check whether or not you have overcrowded the ingredients. This is the main reason why food might not cook evenly in an air fryer.

2. White smoke: White smoke is usually the result of grease, so make sure that you have added some water to the bottom drawer to prevent the grease from overheating.

3. Black smoke: Black smoke is usually due to burnt food. You need to clean the air fryer after every use. If you do not, then the remaining food particles are burned when you use the appliance again. Turn the machine off and cool it completely. Then check it for burned food.

4. The appliance won't stop: The fan of the air fryer operates at high speed and needs some time to stop. Do not worry, it will stop soon.

Chapter 3. How To Set Times And Temperatures Correctly.

It is essential to read your manufacturer's time and temperature instructions and then, you can adjust both to fit the recipe in question to ensure that you have well-cooked meals. Also, work with a food thermometer to aid you in reaching the accurate internal temperature of meats and seafood for safe consumption.

Vegetables

	Temp (°F)	Time (mins)		Temp (°F)	Time (mins)
Asparagus (1-inch slices)	400 °F	5	Onions (quartered)	400 °F	11
Beets (whole)	400 °F	40	Parsnips (½-inch chunks)	380 °F	15
Bell Peppers (1-inch chunks)	400 °F	15	Pearl Onions	400 °F	10
Broccoli (florets)	400 °F	6	Potatoes (whole baby pieces)	400 °F	15
Broccoli Rabe (chopped)	400 °F	6	Potatoes (1-inch chunks)	400 °F	12
Brussel Sprouts (halved)	380 °F	15	Potatoes (baked whole)	400 °F	40

Vegetable	Temp	Time	Vegetable	Temp	Time
Cabbage (diced)	380 °F	15	Pumpkin (½-inch chunks)	380 °F	13
Carrots (halved)	380 °F	15	Radishes	380 °F	15
Cauliflower (florets)	400 °F	12	Squash (½-inch chunks)	400 °F	12
Collard Greens	250 °F	12	Sweet Potato (baked)	380 °F	30 to 35
Corn on the cob	390 °F	6	Tomatoes (halves)	350 °F	10
Cucumber (½-inch slices)	370 °F	4	Tomatoes (cherry)	400 °F	4
Eggplant (2-inch cubes)	400 °F	15	Turnips (½-inch chunks)	380 °F	15
Fennel (quartered)	370 °F	15	Zucchini (½-inch sticks)	400 °F	12
Green Beans	400 °F	5	Mushrooms (¼-inch slices)	400 °F	5
Kale (halved)	250 °F	12			

Chicken

	Temp (°F)	Time (mins)		Temp (°F)	Time (mins)
Breasts, bone in (1 ¼ lb.)	370 °F	25	**Legs, bone-in (1 ¾ lb.)**	380 °F	30
Breasts, boneless (4 oz)	380 °F	12	**Thighs, boneless (1 ½ lb.)**	380 °F	18 to 20
Drumsticks (2 ½ lb.)	370 °F	20	**Wings (2 lb.)**	400 °F	12
Game Hen (halved 2 lb.)	390 °F	20	**Whole Chicken**	360 °F	75
Thighs, bone-in (2 lb.)	380 °F	22	**Tenders**	360 °F	8 to 10

Beef

	Temp (°F)	Time (mins)		Temp (°F)	Time (mins)
Beef Eye Round Roast (4 lb.s.)	400 °F	45 to 55	**Meatballs (1-inch)**	370 °F	7
Burger Patty (4 oz.)	370 °F	16 to 20	**Meatballs (3-inch)**	380 °F	10

Filet Mignon (8 oz.)	400 °F	18	Ribeye, bone-in (1-inch, 8 oz)	400 °F	10 to 15
Flank Steak (1.5 lb.s)	400 °F	12	Sirloin steaks (1-inch, 12 oz)	400 °F	9 to 14
Flank Steak (2 lb.s)	400 °F	20 to 28			

Pork & Lamb

	Temp (°F)	Time (mins)		Temp (°F)	Time (mins)
Bacon (regular)	400 °F	5 to 7	Pork Tenderloin	370 °F	15
Bacon (thick cut)	400 °F	6 to 10	Sausages	380 °F	15
Pork Loin (2 lb.)	360 °F	55	Lamb Loin Chops (1-inch thick)	400 °F	8 to 12
Pork Chops, bone in (1-inch, 6.5 oz)	400 °F	12	Rack of Lamb (1.5 – 2 lb.)	380 °F	22

Fish & Seafood

	Temp (°F)	Time (mins)		Temp (°F)	Time (mins)
Calamari (8 oz)	400 °F	4	**Tuna Steak**	400 °F	7 to 10
Fish Fillet (1-inch, 8 oz)	400 °F	10	**Scallops**	400 °F	5 to 7
Salmon, fillet (6 oz)	380 °F	12	**Shrimp**	400 °F	5
Swordfish steak	400 °F	10			

Frozen Foods

	Temp (°F)	Time (mins)		Temp (°F)	Time (mins)
Breaded Shrimp	400 °F	9	**French Fries (thick - 17 oz)**	400 °F	18
Chicken Nuggets (12 oz)	400 °F	10	**Mozzarella Sticks (11 oz)**	400 °F	8
Fish Sticks (10 oz.)	400 °F	10	**Onion Rings (12 oz)**	400 °F	8
Fish Fillets (½-inch, 10 oz)	400 °F	14	**Pot Stickers (10 oz)**	400 °F	8
French Fries (thin - 20 oz)	400 °F	14			

Converting Recipes

Take your favorite traditional method recipes and convert them over to amazing air frying creations. Virtually anything you have a recipe to cook in the oven, you can convert to cook in the air fryer. Remember the air fryer heat is significantly more intense than a standard oven so start by reducing the suggested temperature by 25°F to 50°F and reduce the time approximately 20%.

If the recipe calls for something to be baked at 425°F for 60 minutes you would air fry it at 400°F for 48 minutes, timing may vary. Always feel free to open the air fryer and check for doneness.

Cooking packaged foods can also apply to the same rules as above. For example, if you are cooking frozen fries, the bag suggests 450°F for 18 minutes then cook the fries at 400°F for 15 minutes. Remember to shake the basket with items like French fries to help with the cooking process and evenly browning.

Chapter 4. How To Clean The Inside Of The Air Fryer.

Air Fryer - Cleaning & Maintenance

The first thing you should have at your fingertips is that, if you do not clean and maintain your air fryer from time to time, it won't last long. Following these guidelines will secure the fact that your air fryer will remain effective and durable for years to come

How To Clean Your Air Fryer:

1. Unplug your air fryer from the wall socket and allow it to cool until you can touch.

2. Using a wet rag, wipe the exterior part of your air fryer

3. Remove the air fryer pan, tray, basket and wash it with hot water and a dishwasher soap in your sink. These parts are removable and are safe for an easy cleanup.

4. Use a cloth or sponge to wipe and clean the inner part of your air fryer

5. If you find any ingredients sticking in your air fryer, scrub it off with a brush.

6. Before adding the pan, tray, and basket back into your air fryer ensure they are entirely dry

7. Once your air fryer is cleaned, store it safely.

How To Maintain Your Air Fryer:

Your air fryer requires a standard form of maintenance to ensure it does not get damaged or work erroneously. To do this, one needs to follow this instruction

1. Before using your air fryer, make sure you check the cord. That is, do not plug a damaged cord into an outlet; this can result in a ghastly injury or even death.

2. Make sure your air fryer is clean and free of any debris before you begin cooking. Check the inner part and make sure you remove anything redundant in there.

3. Ensure the air fryer is placed upright, on a flat surface.

4. Make sure that your air fryer is not too close to the wall or another appliance. Air fryers require 4-inches of space all around them.

5. One after the other, check each component of your air fryer, including the basket, pan, and handle.

6. If you find anything damaged or wrong with your air fryer, reach the manufacturer and get it replaced.

Cleaning Your Air Fryer

1. Unplug the appliance and let it cool down.

2. Wipe the outside with a damp cloth.

3. Wash the basket, tray, and pan with hot water and soap. You can also use a dishwasher to wash these parts.

4. Clean the inside of the air fryer with a damp cloth or sponge.

5. Clean any food that is stuck to the heating element.

6. Dry the parts and assemble the air fryer.

Tips:

1. Use damp cloths to remove stuck-on food. Do not use utensils to avoid scratching the non-stick coating.

2. If the stuck-on food has hardened onto the basket or pan, then soak them in hot soapy water before trying to remove them.

Safety Tips

1. Do not buy a cheap, low-quality air fryer.

2. Do not place it on an uneven surface.

3. Do not overcrowd the basket.

4. Do not leave the appliance unattended.

5. Read the air fryer manual before using it.

6. Clean the appliance after every use.

7. Do not wash the electrical components.

8. Use the right amount of oil. Your air fryer needs only a little oil, so do not use extra.

9. Grease the air fryer basket. It will prevent food from getting stuck and prevent potential burning and smoking.

10. Dry your hands before touching the air fryer.

11. Make sure accessories are air fryer safe.

12. Shake the basket or flip the food during the middle of the cooking to ensure even cooking.

13. If your air fryer needs repairing, seek professional support.

Cleaning Your Air Fryer

It is crucial to maintain your air fryer, and you should clean it regularly to make sure it continues to work to the best of its availability. Below, we will show you what to do.

First, unplug your air fryer and let it cool before trying to clean it. Rub the outside with a built-in fagor fryer with a damp cloth.

The parts of the balay that are built into the air fryer are made of non-stick coating, so it is not necessary to clean them. However, if the food is stuck to the surface, it is recommended to soak it before washing.

1. How do I clean the metal utensils of a fryer?

Metal utensils should not be used when cleaning the air fryer, as it causes scratches and marks. Instead, you should use a non-abrasive sponge. Clean the pan, tray, and basket with warm water and dish soap. As all removable components are safe for essential dishwasher fryers, you can place them in the dishwasher to wash them. Use liquid soap degreaser for cleaning.

2. How do you clean the inside of the fryer?

It is essential to understand that the inner side of the airtight fryer may require a different type of cleaning. You can clean the inside with warm water and a sponge or cloth. Clean any food that is near the burner or that is above the food basket with a brush. You can use a filter to eliminate odors that are released. Remember to rinse the fryer regularly.

3. What should you do after cleaning?

Make sure that the tray and basket dry thoroughly before putting it back in the fryer. If the fryer has a persistent smell of food, clean it immediately. Even after cleaning, if there is still a smell, soak the pot and basket in a solution of liquid soap up to an hour before rinsing it again.

4. What should you do if the smell does not disappear?

Despite this, if the smell persists, you can cut a lemon in half and rub on the pan and basket or even squirt lemon juice on a paper towel and clean the fryer with it. After half an hour you can rewash. If white smoke comes out of the tray, this implies that there is too much grease on the bottom and that it is breaking due to the heat. Therefore, it needs to be cleaned well.

All these steps will be of great help for the air fryer to work correctly for a long time.

Maintenance and Cleaning of The Product

Air Fryer Maintenance

Beyond regularly cleanings, your air fryer requires some basic maintenance to make sure that it doesn't get damaged or start functioning incorrectly. This includes

1. Making sure the unit is clean and free of any debris before you start cooking. If it has been a long time since you last used your air fryer, check inside. Some dust may have accumulated. If there is any food residue on the basket for pan, clean it out before you start cooking

2. Inspecting the cords before each use. Never plug a damaged or frayed cord into an outlet. It can cause serious injury or even death. Make sure the cords are clean and damage-free before using your air fryer

3. Make sure the air fryer is not placed close to a wall or another appliance. Air fryers need at least 4 inches of space behind them and 4 inches of space above them in order to adequately vent steam and hot air while cooking. Placing them in an enclosed space may cause the fryer to overheat

4. Make sure the air fryer is placed upright, on a level surface, before you start cooking.

5. Visually inspect each component, including the basket, pan and handle prior to each use. If you find any damaged components, contact the manufacturer and get them replaced

Tips on Cleaning

Cleaning the air fryer is easy and it does not require you to do a lot of complicated tasks. The first thing that you need to do is to unplug the air fryer before cleaning to prevent electrocution. The basket is dishwasher-friendly, so you can take it out from the fryer's chamber and clean them in the sink or in the dishwasher.

Once you remove the fryer basket, give extra attention to the base of the fryer where most of the drippings from the food have collected and dried. Make sure that you remove the browning that has accumulated at the base as this can lead to burning in future cooking. You can remove the browning by spraying it with warm soapy water and allowing it to soak for at least an hour. This will soften the browning, so you can easily wipe it clean.

Aside from taking care of the inside of the air fryer, it is also important to clean the exterior using a warm moist cloth.

Chapter 5. Tricks To Better Use The Air Fryer.

Useful Tips and Tricks

Experiment with the functions. Your instant pot does so many things, don't just use it for pressure cooking and get other pots and gadgets for the rest. Otherwise what's the point in having it? Use it to shallow fry, boil, steam, bake, etc. The possibilities are plentiful.

Measure your liquids carefully. Your instant pot has two different limits: the pressure limit and the slow cooker limit. Do not exceed the fluid amount for either! Always count things that liquefy, like gelatine or sugar, as a liquid.

Watch out about overfilling. Your instant pot should not be completely filled. Ever! You need space for pressure and/or steam to build up. Whether you are filling it with food or fluid, always make sure there is plenty of space from the top.

Be careful handling steam. Steam and pressure are nothing to joke around with! Never put your hand right in the steam, and always release the pressure according to the instructions manual. Always seal your instant pot properly before building pressure. Always open it when it is ready

Clean it well after each use. Your instant pot will not last if it ends up with a built up film of fat or layer of burnt and sticky food in it. Besides, that is unhealthy. Even if you have "only" used it to steam, remember that steam carries fat particles and creates a greasy film, so it still needs cleaning

Don't Use quick release unless specified. The pressure that can build up in your instant pot is intense. If you release it too fast you could get hurt. Only use quick release when a recipe specifically calls for it.

Don't Fill it with hot oil. This is not a deep fat fryer! Filling it with oil is dangerous and could cause a grease fire. At the very least, you will break your instant pot.

Don't Try and force it open. Again: intense pressure. Forcing it open could cause a seriously painful blast.

Don't Put things in in huge pieces. Even cooking is important, and big pieces do not respond as well to pressure or quick cooking. Leave the whole chickens for slow cooking only

Do not leave the house when it is on. Unlike with a traditional slow cooker, the instant pot reaches high temperatures, can carry a high voltage, and involves literal pressure

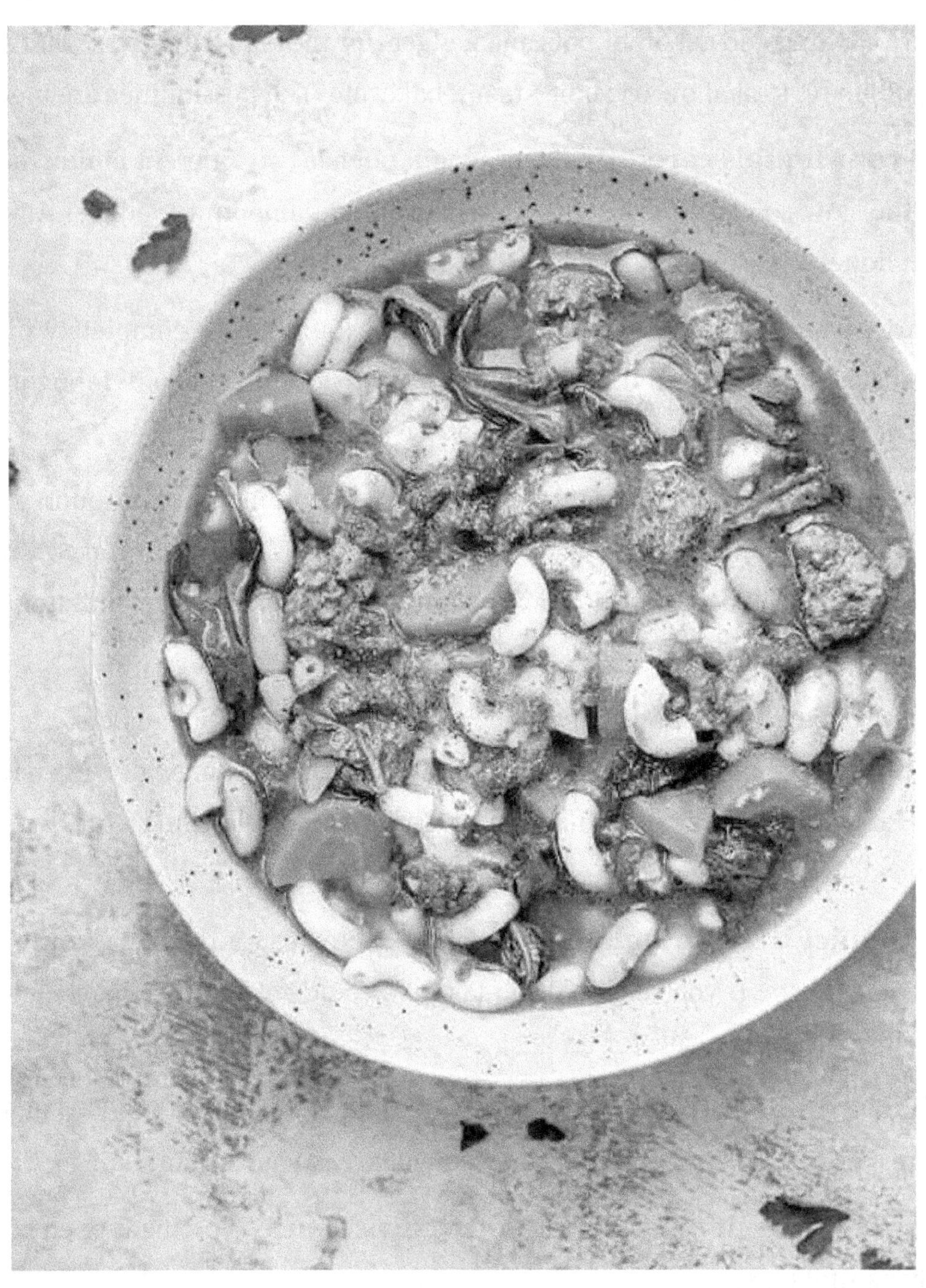

General Air Frying Tips

The following tips are ways to get the most from your air fryer and help you incorporate it into an everyday use appliance.

Tip 1: Placement of your air fryer is important; be sure it is placed on a heat-resistant countertop allowing five inches of space on all sides of the air fryer. This is to allow for proper venting of your air fryer during cooking.

Tip 2: Pre-Heat! Always before frying, bring your basket and inside of the air fryer up to temp. This is simple to do just set your air fryer to the desired temperature and then turn it on for 3 minutes. When the timer sounds, the fryer is heated and you are ready to cook.

Tip 3: Invest in a hand pump kitchen spray bottle. This is a must-have when air frying. While you can brush or drizzle oil onto your food, a spray bottle gives more even coverage. Why not just use spray cans? The spray cans contain different aerosol agents that could break down the non-stick surface of your air fryer. With the hand-pump bottle, you can feel comfortable to spray right inside your basket and give your food the perfect coating.

Tip 4: What's fried food without breading? While you don't have to add breading to some items like chicken wings, there are many that like to. The key to breading in your air fryer is being diligent and not skipping steps. Always coat food with flour first, then egg then breadcrumbs. Paying close attention to ensure that the breadcrumbs are pressed into the food. The air fryer is a convection oven so it has a really powerful fan and if the bread crumb hasn't adhered well they will come off.

Tip 5: Overcrowding is not good. It is really tempting to toss a few extra in, but when doing this it makes it so that the air cannot fully circulate around what you are cooking. Overcrowding will also make the process take more time.

Tip 6: Use a little water in the bottom under the basket when cooking bacon or other fatty foods. This helps prevent the grease from getting too hot and smoking. Just enough water to slightly cover the bottom but not so much it's coming up into the basket.

Tip 7: Use toothpicks to hold food in place. Light foods sometimes can fly around inside the air fryer. Using a toothpick to hold the bread on top of your grilled cheese sandwich, so it stays in place.

Tip 8: Always remove the basket from the drawer. If you pull the drawer and basket from the air fryer the grease and drippings are still at the bottom of the drawer. Removing the basket allows you to not include any unwanted grease on the plate before serving.

Tip 9: Clean up. Just like any other kitchen appliance, it is important to clean up the basket after every use. This will help keep the basket in good condition and the fried smell out of your kitchen.

Tip 10: Self-drying – Use the air fryer to dry itself; it will work better than any towel in the kitchen. Simply just set the fryer to 300 and turn it on for 3 minutes.

Tips for Using Your air Fryer

1. **Preheat Your Air Fryer**... for a proper, it a normal practice that any cooking item should be preheated. Most air fryers recommend that the air fryer should be preheated to ensure even cooking. Often I do it, sometimes I don't do it, and my meal is still good. And in case your air fryer is without preheat feature, simply turn it to the desired temperature and allow it to run for about 3 minutes before bringing adding the food.

2. **Use Oil For Foods Cooked In The Air Fryer**... I like using oils for certain foods to make them crisp, but some foods don't always need it. If your diet has some fat on it (dark meat chicken, ground beef, fatty cuts of meat, etc.) so you really don't

need oil. I use vegetable oil (like my Breakfast Air Fried Potatoes) and any dried seafood, Like the Crispy Air Fryer Fish).

3. **Grease Your Air Fryer**: Container Even if your food does not need oil, do take a moment to at least grease your air frier container. I grease mine by rubbing or brushing a little bit of oil on the bottom of the grates. This will make sure the diet isn't going to stay on it.

4. **Never Use Aerosol Spray Cans In The Air Fryer**: The Aerosol spray cans (such as Pam and related brands) are known to cause chipping in many Air Fryer containers. The aerosol cans contain toxic chemicals that don't match with the covering on most of the containers.

5. **Don't Overload The Basket**: If you want your fried food to turn out to be fresh, you'll want to make sure you don't congest the refrigerator. Placing too much food in the bowl will keep the food from stretching and browning. Cook your food in containers or invest in a larger air fryer to make sure this doesn't happen.

6. **Shake The Basket During Frying, Wings And Other Cooking**. When frying small items such as chicken wings and French fries, shake the basket every few minutes to ensure uniform cooking, sometimes, instead of throwing, use a pair of silicone kitchen pins to flip over larger items

7. When you open the basket to shake, the air fryer will stop for a while, but it will continue frying the food at the same temperature when you return to the container.

8. **Spray Halfway Through Cooking**: I find that spraying oil halfway through cooking is best done on most foods. I tend to wait to spray halfway through cooking unless it's an element that doesn't need to be sprayed like fatty meats. Coated food items are to be sprayed. Additionally, spray some dried flour spots that still surface halfway through the rain.

9. **Water / Bread In The Base Stops White Smoke**: If it is time to fry a greasy food in your air fryer, don't be shocked to see some white smoke pouring out of the

machine. To solve the problem, just dump a little (about 2Tbsp) of water in the bottom of the container, The smoke stops and the food continues to cook.

Some people place a slice of bread at the bottom of the unit to blot the grease when preparing items that can spread large amounts of grease, such as bacon.

10. **Lookout For The Small Light Items In The Air Fryer**: most of the Air Fryer unit have a powerful fan at the top of the unit. This causes some lighter weighted items to get swept up in the fan, which could be dangerous. I tried to make fried egg roll wrappers once, and it was almost a tragedy. I'm hoping to try it again once I figured out how to stop flying around.

11. **Adjust The Temperature**: Most times you want to turn the heat of the Air Fryer to the highest temperature to encourage it to work, but be careful as some foods will dry out easily. A proper way is to adjust the temperature and time from how long you would usually do it in the oven. I like to go down 30 degrees and cut the time by about 20 percent. For starters, if you baked brownies at 350 degrees Fahrenheit in the oven for 20 minutes, cut the Air Fryer to 320 degrees and cook for about 16 minutes.

12. **Invest In The Best Fast Read Thermometer**: Having a good quality quick read thermometer is of the utmost importance when it comes to cooking those meats in your Air Fryer, such as fish, chicken and pork.

Step-By-Step Air Frying

Air fryers work on Rapid Air Technology. The cooking chamber of the air fryer emits heat from a heating element that is close to the food. The exhaust fan that is present above the cooking chamber aids in the necessary airflow from the underside. For cooking using an air fryer, here are some steps that you need to follow:

Prepare Fried Foods:

- Place the air fryer on a level and heatproof kitchen top.

- Prepare the foods.

- Grease the basket with a little oil and add a bit more to the food to avoid sticking.

- If the food is marinated, pat it dry lightly to prevent splattering and excess smoke.

- Use aluminum foil for easy cleaning.

Before Cooking:

- Preheat the air fryer for 3 minutes before cooking.

- Avoid overcrowding and leave sufficient space for air circulation.

During Cook Time:

- Add water into the air fryer drawer to prevent excessive smoke and heat

- Shake the basket or flip the food for even cooking at the halfway mark.

After Cooking:

- Remove the basket from the drawer before taking out the food.

- The juices in the air fryer drawer can be used to make delicious marinades and sauces

- Unplug, cool, and then clean both the basket and drawer after use

250 HEALTHY AND TASTY RECIPES:

Chapter 6. Easy Breakfast

Asparagus Omelet

Cooking Time: 8 minutes

Servings: 2

Ingredients:

3 eggs

5 steamed asparagus tips

2 tablespoons of warm milk

1 tablespoon parmesan cheese, grated

Salt and pepper to taste

Non-stick cooking spray

Directions:

Mix in a large bowl, eggs, cheese, milk, salt and pepper then blend them. Spray a baking pan with non-stick cooking spray. Pour the egg mixture into pan and add the asparagus then place pan inside of baking basket. Set air fryer to 320°Fahrenheit for 8-minutes. Serve warm.

Nutrition: Calories: 231, Total Fat: 9.2g, Carbs: 8g, Protein: 12.2g

Air Baked Eggs

Cooking Time: 8 minutes

Servings: 4

Ingredients:

1 lb. of spinach, chopped

7 ounces sliced ham

4 eggs

1 tablespoon olive oil

4 tablespoons milk

Salt and pepper to taste

Directions:

Preheat your air fryer to 300°Fahrenheit for a cook time of 10-minutes. Butter the inside of 4 ramekins. In each ramekin, place spinach on bottom, one egg, 1 tablespoon of milk, salt, and pepper. Place ramekins in air fryer basket and cook for 8-minutes.

Nutrition: Calories: 213, Total Fat: 9.2g, Carbs: 8.4g, Protein: 13.2g

Pumpkin Pie French Toast

Cooking Time: 20 minutes

Servings: 4

Ingredients:

2 large, beaten eggs

4 slices of cinnamon swirl bread

¼ cup milk

¼ cup pumpkin purée

¼ teaspoon pumpkin spices

¼ cup butter

Directions:

In a large mixing bowl, mix milk, eggs, pumpkin purée and pie spice. Whisk until mixture is smooth. In the egg mixture dip the bread on both sides. Place rack inside of air fryer's cooking basket. Place 2 slices of bread onto rack. Set the temperature to 340°Fahrenheit for 10-minutes. Serve pumpkin pie toast with butter.

Nutrition: Calories: 212, Total Fat: 8.2g, Carbs: 7g, Protein: 11.3g

Air Fryer Scrambled Egg

Cooking Time: 10 minutes

Servings: 2

Ingredients:

2 eggs

1 tomato, chopped

Dash of salt

1 teaspoon butter

¼ cup cream

Directions:

In a bowl, whisk the eggs, salt, and cream until fluffy. Preheat air fryer to 300°Fahrenheit. Add butter to baking pan and place into preheated air fryer. Once the butter is melted, add the egg mixture to baking pan and tomato then cook for 10-minutes. Whisk the eggs until fluffy then serve warm.

Nutrition: Calories: 105, Total Fat: 8g, Carbs: 2.3g, Protein: 6.4g

Breakfast Cheese Bread Cups

Cooking Time: 15 minutes

Servings: 2

Ingredients:

2 eggs

2 tablespoons cheddar cheese, grated

Salt and pepper to taste

1 ham slice, cut into 2 pieces

4 bread slices, flatten with rolling pin

Directions:

Spray the inside of 2 ramekins with cooking spray. Place 2 flat pieces of bread into each ramekin. Add the ham slice pieces into each ramekin. Crack an egg in each ramekin then sprinkle with cheese. Season with salt and pepper. Place the ramekins into air fryer at 300°Fahrenheit for 15-minutes. Serve warm.

Nutrition: Calories: 162, Total Fat: 8g, Carbs: 10g, Protein: 11g

Breakfast Cod Nuggets

Cooking Time: 10 minutes

Servings: 4

Ingredients:

1 lb. of cod

For breading:

2 eggs, beaten

2 tablespoons olive oil

1 cup almond flour

¾ cup breadcrumbs

1 teaspoon dried parsley

Pinch of sea salt

½ teaspoon black pepper

Directions:

Preheat the air fryer to 390°Fahrenheit. Cut the cod into strips about 1-inch by 2-inches in length. Blend breadcrumbs, olive oil, salt, parsley and pepper in a food processor. In three separate bowls add breadcrumbs, eggs, and flour. Place each piece of fish into flour, then the eggs and lastly the breadcrumbs. Add pieces of cod to air fryer basket and cook for 10-minutes. Serve warm.

Nutrition: Calories: 213, Total Fat: 12.6g, Carbs: 9.2g, Protein: 13.4g

Vegetable Egg Pancake

Cooking Time: 15 minutes

Servings: 2

Ingredients:

1 cup almond flour

½ cup milk

1 tablespoon parmesan cheese, grated

3 eggs

1 potato, grated

1 beet, peeled and grated

1 carrot, grated

1 zucchini, grated

1 tablespoon olive oil

¼ teaspoon nutmeg

1 teaspoon onion powder

1 teaspoon garlic powder

½ teaspoon black pepper

Directions:

Preheat your air fryer to 390 ° Fahrenheit. Mix the zucchini, potato, beet, carrot, eggs, milk, almond flour and parmesan in bowl. Place olive oil into oven-safe dish. Form patties with vegetable mix and flatten to form patties. Place patties into oven-safe dish and cook in air fryer for 15-minutes. Serve with sliced tomatoes, sour cream, and toast.

Nutrition: Calories: 223, Total Fat: 11.2g, Carbs: 10.3g, Proteins: 13.4g

Oriental Omelet

Cooking Time: 12 minutes

Servings: 1

Ingredients:

½ cup fresh Shimeji mushrooms, sliced

2 eggs, whisked

Salt and pepper to taste

1 clove of garlic, minced

A handful of sliced tofu

2 tablespoons onion, finely chopped

Cooking spray

Directions:

Spray baking dish with cooking spray. Add onions and garlic. Air fry in preheated air fryer at 355°Fahrenheit for 4-minutes. Place the tofu and mushrooms over the onions and add salt and pepper to taste. Whisk the eggs and pour them over tofu and mushrooms. Air fry again for 20-minutes. Serve warm.

Nutrition: Calories: 210, Total Fat: 11.2g, Carbs: 8.6g, Protein: 12.2g

Crispy Breakfast Avocado Fries

Cooking Time: 8 minutes

Servings: 2

Ingredients:

2 eggs, beaten

2 large avocados, peeled, pitted, cut into 8 slices each

¼ teaspoon pepper

½ teaspoon cayenne pepper

Salt to taste

Juice of ½ a lemon

½ cup of whole wheat flour

1 cup whole wheat breadcrumbs

Greek yogurt to serve

Directions:

Add flour, salt, pepper and cayenne pepper to bowl and mix. Add bread crumbs into another bowl. Beat eggs in a third bowl. First, dredge the avocado slices in the flour mixture. Next, dip them into the egg mixture and finally dredge them in the breadcrumbs. Place avocado fries into the air fryer basket. Preheat the air fryer to 390°Fahrenheit. Place the air fryer basket into the air fryer and cook for 6-minutes. When cook time is completed, transfer the avocado fries onto a serving platter. Sprinkle with lemon juice and serve with Greek yogurt.

Nutrition: Calories: 272, Total Fat: 13.4g, Carbs: 11.2g, Protein: 15.4g

Cheese & Egg Breakfast Sandwich

Cooking Time: 6 minutes

Servings: 1

Ingredients:

1-2 eggs

1-2 slices of cheddar or Swiss cheese

A bit of butter

1 roll sliced in half (your choice, Kaiser bun, English muffin, etc.

Directions:

Butter your sliced roll on both sides. Place the eggs in an oven-safe dish and whisk. Add seasoning if you wish such as dill, chives, oregano, and salt. Place the egg dish, roll and cheese into the air fryer. Make sure the buttered sides of roll are facing upwards. Set the air fryer to 390°Fahrenheit with a cook time of 6-minutes. Remove the ingredients when cook time is completed by air fryer. Place the egg and cheese between the pieces of roll and serve warm. You might like to try adding slices of avocado and tomatoes to this breakfast sandwich!

Nutrition: Calories: 212, Total Fat: 11.2g, Carbs: 9.3g, Protein: 12.4g

Breakfast Zucchini & Cream Muffins

Cook Time: 15 minutes

Servings: 5

Ingredients:

1 tablespoon cream cheese

Half a cup zucchini, shredded

1 tablespoon plain yogurt

1 egg

1 cup of milk

2 tablespoons of warmed coconut oil

Pinch of sea salt

2 teaspoons baking powder

1 teaspoon cinnamon

1 tablespoon liquid Stevia

4 cups whole wheat flour

Directions:

Mix all your dry ingredients in a mixing bowl (flour, sea salt, baking powder and cinnamon. Stir to combine. In another mixing bowl combine all of the wet ingredients (coconut oil, milk, yogurt, liquid Stevia, and egg. Whisk these until evenly combined. In a large bowl combine both the wet and dry ingredients and use a hand mixer to whisk them. Stir in the shredded zucchini and fold in the cream cheese. Place five muffin cups into your air fryer. Fill each cup ¾ full of mixture. Set air fryer to 350°Fahrenheit and cook muffins for 12-minutes. Serve warm or cold.

Nutrition: Calories: 217, Total Fat: 9.3g, Carbs: 8g, Protein: 10.2g

Peanut Butter & Banana Breakfast Sandwich

Cooking Time: 6 minutes

Servings: 1

Ingredients:

2 slices of whole wheat bread

1 teaspoon of sugar-free maple syrup

1 sliced banana

2 tablespoons of peanut butter

Directions:

Evenly coat both sides of the slices of bread with peanut butter. Add the sliced banana and drizzle with some sugar-free maple syrup. Heat in the air fryer to 330°Fahrenheit for 6 minutes. Serve warm.

Nutrition: Calories: 211, Total Fat: 8.2g, Carbs: 6.3g, Protein: 11.2g

Eggs & Cocotte on Toast

Cooking Time: 15 minutes

Servings: 2

Ingredients:

1/8 teaspoon of black pepper

¼ teaspoon salt

½ teaspoon Italian seasoning

¼ teaspoon balsamic vinegar

¼ teaspoon sugar-free maple syrup

1 cup sausages, chopped into small pieces

2 eggs

2 slices of whole wheat toast

3 tablespoons cheddar cheese, shredded

6-slices tomatoes

Cooking spray

A little mayonnaise to serve

Directions:

Spray baking dish with cooking spray. Place the bread slices at the bottom of dish. Sprinkle the sausages over bread. Lay the tomatoes over it. Sprinkle top with cheese. Beat the eggs and then pour over top of bread slices. Drizzle vinegar and maple syrup over eggs. Season with Italian seasoning, salt, and pepper, then sprinkle some more cheese on top. Place the baking dish in the air fryer basket that should be preheated at 320° Fahrenheit and cooked for 10-minutes. Remove from air fryer and add spot of mayonnaise and serve.

Nutrition: Calories: 232, Total Fat: 7.4g, Carbs: 6.3g, Protein: 14.2g

Breakfast Frittata

Cooking Time: 15 minutes

Servings: 3

Ingredients:

6 eggs

8 cherry tomatoes, halved

2 tablespoons parmesan cheese, shredded

1 Italian sausage, diced

Salt and pepper to taste

Directions:

Preheat your air fryer to 355°Fahrenheit. Add the tomatoes and sausage to baking dish. Place the baking dish into air fryer and cook for 5-minutes. Meanwhile, add eggs, salt, pepper, cheese, and oil into mixing bowl and whisk well. Remove the baking dish from air fryer and pour the egg mixture on top, spreading evenly. Placing the dish back into the air fryer and bake for an additional 5-minutes. Remove from air fryer and slice into wedges and serve.

Nutrition: Calories: 273, Total Fat: 8.2g, Carbs: 7g, Protein: 14.2g

Country Breakie Chicken Tenders

Cooking Time: 15 minutes

Servings: 4

Ingredients:

¾ lb. of chicken tenders

For breading:

2 tablespoons olive oil

1 teaspoon black pepper

½ teaspoon salt

½ cup seasoned breadcrumbs

½ cup all-purpose flour

2 eggs, beaten

Directions:

Preheat your air fryer to 330°Fahrenheit. In three separate bowls, set aside breadcrumbs, eggs, and flour. Season the breadcrumbs with salt and pepper. Add olive oil to the breadcrumbs and mix well. Place chicken tenders into flour, then dip into eggs and finally dip into breadcrumbs. Press to ensure that the breadcrumbs are evenly coating the chicken. Shake off excess breading in cooking basket. Cook the chicken tenders for 10-minutes in the air fryer. Serve warm.

Nutrition: Calories: 276, Total Fat: 8.6g, Carbs: 7g, Protein: 13.2g

Baked Mini Quiche

Cooking Time: 15 minutes

Servings: 2

Ingredients:

2 eggs

1 large yellow onion, diced

1 ¾ cups whole wheat flour

1 ½ cups spinach, chopped

¾ cup cottage cheese

Salt and black pepper to taste

2 tablespoons olive oil

¾ cup butter

¼ cup milk

Directions:

Preheat the air fryer to 355°Fahrenheit. Add the flour, butter, salt, and milk to bowl and knead dough until smooth and refrigerate for 15-minutes. Place a frying pan over medium heat and add the oil to it. When the oil is heated, add the onions into pan and sauté them. Add spinach to pan and cook until it wilts. Drain excess moisture from spinach. Whisk the eggs together and add cheese to bowl and mix. Take the dough out of the fridge and divide into 8 equal parts. Roll the dough into a round that will fit into bottom of quiche mold. Place the rolled dough into molds. Place the spinach filling over dough. Place molds into air fryer basket and place basket inside of air fryer and cook for 15-minutes. Remove quiche from molds and serve warm or cold.

Nutrition: Calories: 262, Total Fat: 8.2g, Carbs: 7.3g, Protein: 9.5g

Morning Mini Cheeseburger Sliders

Cooking Time: 10 minutes

Servings: 6

Ingredients:

1 lb. ground beef

6 slices of cheddar cheese

6 dinner rolls

Salt and black pepper to taste

Directions:

Preheat your air fryer to 390°Fahrenheit. Form 6 beef patties each about 2.5 ounces and season with salt and black pepper. Add the burger patties to the cooking basket and cook them for 10-minutes. Remove the burger patties from the air fryer; place the cheese on top of burgers and return to air fryer and cook for another minute. Remove and put burgers on dinner rolls and serve warm.

Nutrition: Calories: 262, Total Fat: 9.4g, Carbs: 8.2g, Protein: 16.2g

Avocado & Blueberry Muffins

Cooking Time: 15 minutes

Servings: 12

Ingredients:

2 eggs

1 cup blueberries

2 cups almond flour

1 teaspoon baking soda

1/8 teaspoon salt

2 ripe avocados, peeled, pitted, mashed

2 tablespoons liquid Stevia

1 cup plain Greek yogurt

1 teaspoon vanilla extract

For streusel topping:

2 tablespoons Truvia sweetener

4 tablespoons butter, softened

4 tablespoons almond flour

Directions:

Make the streusel topping by mixing Truvia, flour, and butter until you form a crumbly mixture. Place this mixture in the freezer for a while. Meanwhile, make the muffins by sifting together flour, baking powder, baking soda and salt and set aside. Add avocados and liquid Stevia to a bowl and mix well. Adding in one egg at a time, continue to beat. Add the vanilla extract and yogurt and beat again. Add in flour mixture a bit at a time and mix well. Add the blueberries into mixture and gently fold them in. Pour the batter into greased muffin cups, then add mixture until they are half-full. Sprinkle the streusel topping mixture on top of muffin mixture and place muffin cups in the air fryer basket.

Bake in preheated air fryer at 355°Fahrenheit for 10-minutes. Remove the muffin cups from the air fryer and allow them to cool. Cool completely then serve.

Nutrition: Calories: 202, Total Fat: 9.2g, Carbs: 7.2g, Protein: 6.3g

Grilled Cheese

Cooking Time: 7 minutes

Servings: 2

Ingredients:

4 slices of brown bread

½ cup sharp cheddar cheese, shredded

¼ cup butter, melted

Directions:

Preheat your air fryer to 360°Fahrenheit. Place cheese and butter into separate bowls. Melt butter and brush it onto the 4 slices of bread. Place cheese on 2 sides of bread slices. Put sandwiches together and place them into cooking basket. Cook in air fryer for 5-minutes and serve warm.

Nutrition: Calories: 214, Total Fat: 11.2g, Carbs: 9.4g, Protein: 13.2g

Breakfast Muffins

Cooking Time: 6 minutes

Servings: 2

Ingredients:

2 whole wheat English muffins

4 slices of bacon

Pepper to taste

2 eggs

Directions:

Crack an egg each into ramekins. Season with pepper. Place the ramekins in your preheated air fryer at 390°Fahrenheit for 6-minutes with the bacon and muffins alongside. Remove the muffins from air fryer after a few minutes and split them. When the bacon and eggs are done cooking, add two pieces of bacon and one egg to each egg muffin and serve immediately.

Nutrition: Calories: 276, Total Fat: 12g, Carbs: 10.2g, Protein: 17.3g

Cheese Omelette

Cooking Time: 15 minutes

Servings: 2

Ingredients:

3 eggs

1 large yellow onion, diced

2 tablespoons cheddar cheese, shredded

½ teaspoon soy sauce

Salt and pepper to taste

Olive oil cooking spray

Directions:

In a bowl whisk together eggs, soy sauce, pepper, and salt. Spray with olive oil cooking spray a small pan that will fit inside of your air fryer. Add onions to the pan and spread them around. Air fry onions for 7-minutes. Pour the beaten egg mixture over the cooked onions and sprinkle the top with shredded cheese. Place back into the air fryer and cook for 6-minutes more. Remove from the air fryer and serve omelet with toasted multi-grain bread.

Nutrition: Calories: 232, Total Fat: 8.2g, Carbs: 6.2g, Protein: 12.3g

Full English Breakfast

Preparation Time: 30 MIN

Servings: 4

Ingredients:

8 Bacon Rashers

8 Sausages

10 oz Canned Baked Beans, drained

8 Medium Eggs

16 Cherry Tomatoes, halved

16 Button Mushrooms halved

Salt to taste

Ground Black Pepper to taste

8 Toast Slices

Directions:

Put sausages and bacon in the Air Fryer, use the grill pan accessory if available, and cook them for 10 minutes at 360 degrees F.

When done transfer them to serving plates.

While sausages and bacon are cooking take four 4 ounces ramekins and crack two eggs in each of them, add salt and pepper to taste.

Pour beans in a 10 ounces ramekin, add salt and pepper.

Place both ramekins with eggs and the one with beans in the Air Fryer and cook for 10 minutes at 400 degrees F.

Remove ramekins from the Air Fryer and place in it mushroom halves and cook them for 6 minutes at 400 degrees F.

Transfer eggs to the plates with bacon and sausages.

Stir beans and then spoon a quarter next to eggs on each plate.

Add the cherry tomatoes to the Air Fryer, sprinkle both mushrooms and tomatoes with salt and pepper to taste and cook for another 4 minutes at 400 degrees F.

Divide tomatoes and mushrooms onto each plate.

Enjoy!

Roasted Baby Potatoes

Preparation Time: 16 MIN

Servings: 4

Ingredients:

1 ½ lbs Baby Potatoes, skinned and quartered

1 Red Bell Pepper, cut into 1-inch cubes

1 Medium Onion, diced

½ tsp Garlic Powder

1 tbsp. Olive oil

1 tsp Rosemary, chopped

Salt to taste

Ground Black Pepper to taste

Directions:

Preheat the Air Fryer to 400 degrees F.

Place all ingredients in a bowl and toss well to combine.

Cook in the Air Fryer for 15 minutes at 400 degrees, shaking twice during the cooking.

Enjoy!

Frittata

Preparation Time: 15 MIN

Servings: 3

Ingredients:

5 Baby Potatoes, cut into ½ inch cubes

1 tbsp. Olive Oil

1 Italian Sausage, cut into 1-inch slices

1 Red Bell Pepper, cut into 1-inch cubes

1 Small Onion, cut into 1-inch cubes

3 eggs

1 tbsp. Parsley Leaves, chopped

1 pinch Garlic Powder

2 tbsp. Grated Parmesan Cheese

Salt to taste

Ground Black Pepper to the taste

Directions:

Place baby potato cubes in the Air Fryer accessory, add the olive oil, salt, and pepper to taste, and toss to mix well.

Cook for 5 minutes at 400 degrees F.

Add the sausage, bell pepper, and onion to the Air Fryer accessory. Toss to mix and cook another 5 minutes at 400 degrees F.

Meanwhile, whisk three eggs and then add to them the parsley, garlic powder, parmesan, and pepper to taste, and stir well to combine.

Pour the egg mixture over potatoes and sausages in the Air Fryer accessory and cook for 10 minutes at 360 degrees F.

Serve warm.

Enjoy!

Baked Spinach and Ham Eggs

Preparation Time: 25 MIN

Servings: 4

Ingredients:

1 lbs Baby Spinach

1 tbsp. olive oil

1 tbsp. Butter, melted and cooled to room temperature

7 oz Ham, grated

4 eggs

4 tbsp. milk

Salt and black pepper to the taste

Directions:

Warm up a pan over medium heat.

Add olive oil and spinach to pan. Toss and sauté for 2 minutes to wilt.

Brush four ramekins with melted butter.

Place a quarter of spinach in each of the ramekins, and add grated ham over it.

Also divide ham in each of the ramekins.

Crack an egg in each ramekin as well and top with the milk.

Season with salt and pepper, place ramekins in your air fryer's basket, cover and cook at 360 degrees F for 20 minutes.

Serve hot for breakfast.

Enjoy!

Cheese and Mushroom Frittata

Preparation Time: 8-10 MIN

Servings: 4

Ingredients:

4 cups Button Mushrooms, cut into ¼ inch slices

1 Large Red Onion, cut into ¼ inch slices

2 tbsp. Olive Oil

1 tsp Garlic, minced

6 Eggs

Salt to taste

Ground Black Pepper to taste

6 tbsp. Feta Cheese

Directions:

Put the button mushrooms, onions and garlic in a pan with a tbsp. of olive oil, and sauté over medium heat for 5 minutes.

Transfer on a kitchen towel to dry and cool.

Preheat the Air Fryer to 330 degrees F.

Place eggs in a bowl and whisk lightly. Season with salt and pepper and then whisk well.

Brush the baking accessory with olive oil

Place sautéed onions and mushrooms in the baking accessory, crumble the feat cheese over it, and then pour the eggs on top.

Cook for 20 minutes or until a skewer stuck in the middle of frittata comes out clean.

Serve warm.

Enjoy!

Banana Flapjacks

Preparation Time: 8-10 MIN

Servings: 2

Ingredients:

1 Large Banana

2 Eggs

Olive Oil for greasing

Directions:

Preheat the Air Fryer to 330 degrees F.

Place in a bowl eggs and whisk them.

Add banana to eggs and lightly mash it with a fork.

Spoon quarters of the mixture in the Air Fryer basket.

Cook for 3 minutes, then flip and cook for another 3 minutes.

Enjoy!

Bagels

Preparation Time: 20 MIN

Servings: 12

Ingredients:

½ lb. flour

1 tsp. active dry yeast

1 tsp. brown sugar

½ cup lukewarm water

2 tbsp. butter softened

1 tsp salt

1 large egg

Directions:

Dissolve the yeast and sugar in the warm water. Let rest for 5 minutes.

Add the remaining ingredients and mix until sticky dough forms. Cover and let rest for 40 minutes.

Knead the dough on a lightly floured surface and divide into 5 large balls. Let rest for 4 minutes.

Preheat air fryer to 360 degrees F.

Flatted the dough balls and make a hole in the center of each. Arrange the bagels on a baking sheet lined with parchment paper. Bake for 20 minutes.

Enjoy!

Creamy and Cheesy Pancake

Preparation Time: 8-10 MIN

Servings: 1

Ingredients:

2 Eggs

1 pack Stevia

½ tsp Cinnamon

2 cups Cream Cheese

Directions:

Preheat the Air Fryer to 330 degrees F.

Place the eggs and stevia in a bowl and whisk until stevia is dissolved.

Add the cinnamon and cream cheese to eggs and whisk until smooth.

Ladle the quarter of batter into Air Fryer accessory and cook for 2 minutes at 330 degrees F.

Flip the pancake and cook for 2 more minutes.

Repeat for the rest of batter.

Enjoy!

Vegetarian Omelet

Preparation Time: 16 MIN

Servings: 2

Ingredients:

8 ounces spinach leaves

3 Spring Onions, cut into 1-inch slices

½ Red Bell Pepper, cut into 1-inch cubes

1 cup Button Mushrooms, cut into ¼ inch slices

½ tsp Ground Turmeric

1 tsp Thyme

1 tsp Kala Namak Salt

½ tsp Ground Black Pepper

1 tsp Minced Garlic

3 tbsp. Olive Oil (extra virgin

2 tbsp. Butter

1 cup Chickpea Flour

1 cup Water

Directions:

In a bowl place spring onions, bell peppers, mushrooms, turmeric, thyme, kala namak salt, ground black pepper, minced garlic and two tbsp. of olive oil. Toss well to combine.

Heat a sauté pan over medium-high heat and tip in the vegetable mixture.

Sauté for 3 minutes frequently tossing.

Add spinach and butter to the pan and sauté for another 3 minutes frequently tossing.

Remove from heat and set aside until needed.

In a bowl place the chickpea flour and water, and whisk to smooth batter.

Grease the Air Fryer accessory with olive oil and pour in the batter.

Cook for 3 minutes at 390 degrees F. Flip and cook for another 3 minutes.

Transfer fried omelet on a serving plate and top with sautéed vegetables.

Serve with salsa on the side.

Enjoy!

Bacon and Cheese Rolls

Preparation Time: 8-10 MIN

Servings: 4

Ingredients:

1 lbs Cheddar Cheese, grated

1 lbs Bacon Rashers

1 8 oz can Pillsbury Crescent Dough

Directions:

Preheat the Air Fryer to 330 degrees F.

Cut the bacon rashers across into ¼ inch strips and mix with the cheddar cheese. Set aside.

Cut the dough sheet to 1 by 1.5 inches pieces.

Place an equal amount of bacon and cheese mixture on center of the dough pieces and pinch corners together to enclose stuffing.

Transfer the parcels in the Air Fry basket and bake for 7 minutes at 330 degrees F.

Increase the temperature to 390 degrees F, and bake for another 3 minutes.

Serve warm.

Enjoy!

Meatballs and Creamy Potatoes

Preparation Time: 45-50 MIN

Servings: 4-6

Ingredients:

12 oz Lean Ground Beef

1 Medium Onion, finely chopped

1 tbsp. Parsley Leaves, finely chopped

½ tbsp. Fresh Thyme Leaves

½ tsp Minced Garlic

2 tbsp. Olive Oil

1 tsp Salt

1 tsp Ground Black Pepper

1 Large Egg

3 tbsp. Bread Crumbs

1 cup Half & Half, or ½ cup Whole Milk and ½ cup Cream mixed together

7 Medium Russet Potatoes

½ tsp Ground Nutmeg

½ cup Grated Gruyere Cheese

Directions:

Place the ground beef, onions, parsley, thyme, garlic, olive oil, salt and pepper, egg and breadcrumbs in a bowl and mix well. Place in refrigerator until needed.

In another bowl place half & half and nutmeg, and whisk to combine.

Peel and wash potatoes, and then slice them thinly, ⅛ to ⅕ of an inch, if needed use a mandolin.

Preheat the Air Fryer to 390 degrees F.

Place potato slices in a bowl with half & half and toss to coat well.

Layer the potato slices in an Air Fryer baking accessory and pour over the leftover half & half.

Bake for 25 minutes at 390 degrees F.

Meanwhile, take the meat mixture out of fridge and shape into inch and half balls.

When potatoes are cooked place meatballs on top of them in one layer and cover with the grated Gruyere.

Cook for another 10 minutes.

Enjoy!

Sweet Potato Fritters

Preparation Time: 6-7 MIN

Servings: 4

Ingredients:

1 can Sweet Potato Puree, 15 oz

½ tsp Minced Garlic

½ cup Frozen Spinach, thawed, finely chopped and drained well

1 Large Leek, minced

1 serving Flax Egg

¼ cup Almond Flour

¼ tsp Sweet Paprika Flakes

1 tsp Kosher Salt

½ tsp Ground White Pepper

Directions:

Preheat the Air Fryer to 330 degrees F.

Place all ingredients in a bowl and mix all well.

Divide into 16 balls and flatten each to no more than an inch thick patty.

Place fritters in the Air Fryer basket and cook for two minutes at 330 degrees F.

Flip and cook for 2 more minutes.

If needed cook in batches.

Enjoy!

Chapter 7. Appetizers

Garlic Kale Chips

Cooking Time: 10 minutes

Servings: 2

Ingredients:

1 tablespoon yeast flakes

Sea salt to taste

1 teaspoon vegan seasoning

4 cups packed kale

2 tablespoons olive oil

1 teaspoon garlic, minced

Directions:

In a bowl, place the oil, the pieces of kale, garlic and the ranch seasoning. Add the yeast and mix well. Dump the coated kale into air fryer basket and cook at 375°Fahrenheit for 5-minutes. Shake after 3-minutes and serve.

Nutrition: Calories: 50, Total Fat: 1.9g, Carbs: 10g, Protein: 46g

Garlic Salmon Balls

Cooking Time: 15 minutes

Servings: 2

Ingredients:

6-ounces of tinned salmon

1 large egg

3 tablespoons olive oil

5 tablespoons wheat germ

½ teaspoon garlic powder

1 tablespoon dill, fresh, chopped

4 tablespoons spring onion, diced

4 tablespoons celery, diced

Directions:

Preheat your air fryer to 370°Fahrenheit. In a large bowl, mix the salmon, the egg, celery, onion, dill, and garlic. Shape the mixture into golf ball size balls and roll them in the wheat germ. In a small pan, warm olive oil over medium-low heat. Add the salmon balls and slowly flatten them. Transfer them to your air fryer and cook for 10-minutes.

Nutrition: Calories: 219, Total Fat: 7.7g, Carbs: 14.8g, Protein: 23.1g

Roasted Vegetables with Paprika

Cooking Time: 10 minutes

Servings: 4

Ingredients:

1 lb. tomatoes

1 lb. green peppers

1 onion

3 cloves garlic

4 boiled eggs

1 tablespoon coriander powder

1 tablespoon lemon juice

2 -ounces of black olives

Salt to taste

1 teaspoon paprika

Directions:

Preheat your air fryer to 300°Fahrenheit. Line peppers, tomatoes, garlic, onion in the air fryer basket. Close lid and cook for 5-minutes, then flip veggies around and cook for another 5-minutes. Remove veggies from air fryer and peel their skin. Place the veggies in a blender and sprinkle with salt, lemon juice, and coriander powder. Blend until smooth. Slice eggs in half. Divide veggie mixture up and top each plate with 1 boiled egg cut in half and sprinkle with paprika and drizzle with oil.

Nutrition: Calories: 80, Total Fat: 6g, Carbs: 8g, Protein: 2g

Onion Rings

Cooking Time: 10 minutes

Servings: 3

Ingredients:

1 onion, cut into slices then separate into rings

1 ½ cups almond flour

¾ cup pork rinds

1 cup milk

1 egg

1 tablespoon baking powder

½ teaspoon salt

Directions:

Preheat your air fryer for 10-minutes. Cut onion into slices then separate into rings. In a bowl, add the flour, baking powder, and salt. Whisk the eggs, and the milk then combines with flour. Gently dip the floured onion rings into the batter to coat them. Spread the pork rinds on a plate and dredge the rings in the crumbs. Place the onion rings in your air fryer and cook for 10-minutes at 360°Fahrenheit.

Nutrition: Calories: 304, Total Fat: 18g, Carbs: 31g, Protein: 38g

Crispy Eggplant Fries

Cooking Time: 12 minutes

Servings: 3

Ingredients:

2 eggplants

¼ cup olive oil

¼ cup almond flour

½ cup water

Directions:

Preheat your air fryer to 390°Fahrenheit. Cut the eggplants into half-inch slices. In a mixing bowl, mix the flour, olive oil, water, and eggplants. Slowly coat the eggplants. Add eggplants to air fryer and cook for 12-minutes. Serve with yogurt or tomato sauce.

Nutrition: Calories: 103, Total Fat: 7.3g, Carbs: 12.3g, Protein: 1.9g

Charred Bell Peppers

Cooking Time: 4 minutes

Servings: 3

Ingredients:

20 bell peppers, sliced and seeded

1 teaspoon olive oil

1 pinch of sea salt

1 lemon

Directions:

Preheat your air fryer to 390°Fahrenheit. Sprinkle the peppers with oil and salt. Cook the peppers in air fryer for 4-minutes. Place peppers in a large bowl, and squeeze lemon juice over the top. Season with salt and pepper.

Nutrition: Calories: 30, Total Fat: 0.25g, Carbs: 6.91g, Protein: 1.28g

Garlic Tomatoes

Cooking Time: 15 minutes

Servings: 4

Ingredients:

3 tablespoons of vinegar

½ teaspoon thyme, dried

4 tomatoes

1 tablespoon olive oil

Salt and black pepper to taste

1 clove of garlic, minced

Directions:

Preheat your air fryer to 390°Fahrenheit. Cut the tomatoes into halves and remove the seeds. Place them in a big bowl and toss with oil, salt, pepper, garlic, and thyme. Place them into air fryer and cook for 15-minutes. Drizzle with vinegar and serve.

Nutrition: Calories: 28.9, Total Fat: 2.4g, Carbs: 2.0g, Protein: 0.4g

Mushroom Stew

Cooking Time: 1 hour and 22 minutes

Servings: 6

Ingredients:

1 lb. of chicken, cubed, boneless, skinless

2 tablespoons of canola oil

1 lb. fresh mushrooms, sliced

1 tablespoon thyme, dried

¾ cup of water

2 tablespoons tomato paste

3 large tomatoes, chopped

4 cloves garlic, minced

1 cup green peppers, sliced

3 cups of zucchini, diced

1 large onion, diced

1 tablespoon basil

1 tablespoon marjoram

1 tablespoon oregano

Directions:

Cut the chicken into cubes. Arrange them in the air fryer basket and pour olive oil over them. Add mushrooms, zucchini, onion, and green pepper. Mix and add in garlic, cook for 2-minutes, then add in tomato paste, water, and seasonings. Lock the air fryer and cook the stew for 50-minutes. Set the heat to 340°Fahrenheit and cook for an additional 20-minutes. Remove from air fryer and transfer into a large pan. Pour in a bit of water and simmer for 10-minutes.

Nutrition: Calories: 53, Total Fat: 3.3g, Carbs: 4.9g, Protein: 2.3g

Cheese & Onion Nuggets

Cooking Time: 12 minutes

Servings: 4

Ingredients:

7-ounces Edam cheese, grated

2 spring onions, diced

1 egg, beaten

1 tablespoon coconut oil

1 tablespoon thyme, dried

Salt and pepper to taste

Directions:

Mix the onion, cheese, coconut oil, salt, pepper, thyme in a bowl. Make 8 small balls and place the cheese in the center. Place in fridge for about an hour. With the use of a pastry brush, carefully brush beaten egg over the nuggets. Cook for 12-minutes in air fryer at 350°Fahrenheit.

Nutrition: Calories: 227, Total Fat: 17.3g, Carbs: 4.5g, Protein: 14.2g

Spiced Nuts

Cooking Time: 10 minutes

Servings: 3 cups

Ingredients:

1 cup almonds

1 cup pecan halves

1 cup cashews

1 egg white, beaten

½ teaspoon cinnamon, ground

Pinch of cayenne pepper

¼ teaspoon cloves, ground

Dash of salt

Directions:

Combine the egg white with spices. Preheat your air fryer to 300°Fahrenheit. Toss the nuts in the spiced mixture. Cook for 25-minutes, stirring several times throughout cooking time.

Nutrition: Calories: 88.4, Total Fat: 7.6g, Carbs: 3.9g, Protein: 2.5g

Keto French Fries

Cooking Time: 20 minutes

Servings: 4Ingredients:

1 large rutabaga, peeled, cut into spears about ¼ inch wide

Salt and pepper to taste

½ teaspoon paprika

2 tablespoons coconut oil

Directions:

Preheat your air fryer to 450°Fahrenheit. Mix the oil, paprika, salt, and pepper. Pour the oil mixture over the fries, making sure all pieces are well coated. Cook in air fryer for 20-minutes or until crispy.

Nutrition: Calories: 113, Total Fat: 7.2g, Carbs: 12.5g, Protein: 1.9g

Fried Garlic Green Tomatoes

Cooking Time: 12 minutes

Servings: 2

Ingredients:

3 green tomatoes, sliced

½ cup almond flour

2 eggs, beaten

Salt and pepper to taste

1 teaspoon garlic, minced

Directions:

Season the tomatoes with salt, garlic and pepper. Preheat your air fryer to 400°Fahrenheit. Dip the tomatoes first in flour then in egg mixture. Spray the tomato rounds with olive oil and place in air fryer basket. Cook for 8-minutes, then flip over and cook for an additional 4-minutes. Serve with zero carb mayonnaise.

Nutrition: Calories: 123, Total Fat: 3.9g, Carbs: 16g, Protein: 8.4g

Garlic Cauliflower Tots

Cooking Time: 20 minutes

Servings: 6

Ingredients:

1 head of cauliflower, chopped in a food processor

½ cup parmesan cheese, grated

Salt and pepper to taste

¼ cup almond flour

2 eggs

1 teaspoon garlic, minced

Directions:

Mix all the ingredients. Shape into tots and spray with olive oil. Preheat your air fryer to 400°Fahrenheit. Cook for 10-minutes on each side.

Nutrition: Calories: 18, Total Fat: 0.6g, Carbs: 1.3g, Protein: 1.8g

Green Onion & Parmesan Tomatoes

Cooking Time: 15 minutes

Servings: 4

Ingredients:

4 large tomatoes, cut in slices

1 tablespoon olive oil

Salt and pepper to taste

½ teaspoon thyme, dried

2 garlic cloves, minced

2 green onions, finely chopped

½ cup parmesan, freshly grated

Directions:

Preheat your air fryer to 390°Fahrenheit. Coat the tomato slices with olive oil, season with garlic, thyme, salt, and pepper. Top with parmesan and chopped green onions. Place tomatoes in air fryer and cook for 15-minutes. Serve on top of crostini or any meat, poultry or fish.

Nutrition: Calories: 69, Total Fat: 3.9g, Carbs: 69g, Protein: 1.6g

Green Bell Peppers with Cauliflower Stuffing

Cooking Time: 20 minutes

Servings: 4

Ingredients:

4 green bell peppers, top cut, deseeded

1 teaspoon lemon juice

2 tablespoons coriander leaves, finely chopped

2 green chilies, finely chopped

2 cups cauliflower, cooked and mashed

2 onions, finely chopped

1 teaspoon cumin seeds

¼ teaspoon turmeric powder

¼ teaspoon chili powder

¼ teaspoon garam masala

Salt to taste

Olive oil as needed

Directions:

In a pan heat the oil and sauté the chilies, onion, and cumin seeds. Add the rest of the ingredients except the bell peppers and mix well. Preheat your air fryer to 390°Fahrenheit for 10-minutes. Brush the green bell peppers with olive oil, inside and out and stuff each pepper with cauliflower mixture. Place them into air fryer and grill for 10-minutes.

Nutrition: Calories: 257, Total Fat: 4.0g, Carbs: 44.8g, Protein: 12.3g

Cheesy Chickpea & Courgette Burgers

Cooking Time: 10 minutes

Servings: 4

Ingredients:

1 can chickpeas (drained

3 tablespoons coriander

1 ounce cheddar cheese, shredded

2 eggs, beaten

1 teaspoon garlic puree

1 zucchini (spiralized

1 red onion, diced

1 teaspoon chili powder

1 teaspoon mixed spice

Salt and pepper to taste

1 teaspoon cumin

Directions:

Mix your ingredients in a mixing bowl. Shape portions of the mixture into burgers. Place in the air fryer at 300°Fahrenheit for 15-minutes.

Nutrition: Calories: 184.8, Total Fat: 10.1g, Carbs: 18.4g, Protein: 13.2g

Spicy Sweet Potatoes

Cooking Time: 23 minutes

Servings: 4

Ingredients:

3 sweet potatoes, peeled and chopped into chips

1 teaspoon chili powder

1 teaspoon paprika

2 tablespoons olive oil

1 tablespoon red wine vinegar

1 tomato, thinly sliced

½ cup tomato sauce

1 onion, peeled and diced

Salt and pepper to taste

1 teaspoon rosemary

1 teaspoon oregano

1 teaspoon mixed spice

2 teaspoons thyme

2 teaspoons coriander

Directions:

Toss the chips in a bowl with olive oil. Add to air fryer and cook for 15-minutes at 360°Fahrenheit. Mix the remaining ingredients in a baking dish. Place the sauce in the air fryer for 8-minutes. Toss the potatoes in the sauce and serve warm.

Nutrition: Calories: 303, Total Fat: 5g, Carbs: 57g, Protein: 8g

Olive, Cheese & Broccoli

Cooking Time: 15 minutes

Servings: 4

Ingredients:

2lbs. broccoli florets

2 tablespoons olive oil

¼ cup parmesan cheese, shaved

2 teaspoons lemon zest, grated

1/3 cup Kalamata olives (halved, pitted

½ teaspoon ground black pepper

1 teaspoon sea salt

Directions:

Boil the water in a pan over medium heat and cook the broccoli for about 4-minutes. Drain. Toss the broccoli with salt, pepper, and olive oil in a bowl. Place in the air fryer and cook at 400°Fahrenheit for 15-minutes. Toss twice during cook time. Move to a dish and toss with lemon zest, cheese, and olives.

Nutrition: Calories: 214, Total Fat: 13.45g, Carbs: 13.22g, Protein: 12.56g

Veggie Mix

Cooking Time: 35 minutes

Servings: 4

Ingredients:

½ lb. carrots, peeled, cubed

6 teaspoons olive oil

½ teaspoon tarragon leaves

½ teaspoon white pepper

Salt to taste

1 lb. yellow squash, chopped into wedges

1 lb. zucchini, chopped into wedges

Directions:

Toss the carrots with 2 teaspoons of olive oil in your air fryer basket. Cook at 400°Fahrenheit for 5-minutes. Toss in the squash and zucchini along with the rest of the oil, salt, and pepper into air fryer. Cook for an additional 30-minutes, tossing twice during cook time. Toss with tarragon and serve.

Nutrition: Calories: 162, Total Fat: 1.2g, Carbs: 30.3g, Protein: 7.5g

Garlic & Cheese Potatoes

Cooking Time: 40 minutes

Servings: 4

Ingredients:

4 Idaho baking potatoes, halved

1 tablespoon garlic powder

Salt to taste

½ cup cheddar cheese, shredded

1 teaspoon parsley

Directions:

Toss all your ingredients in a bowl except cheese. Place potatoes in a baking dish and sprinkle cheese over top of them. Cook for 40-minutes at 390°Fahrenheit.

Nutrition: Calories: 498, Total Fat: 19.09g, Carbs: 67.27g, Protein: 16.5g

Garlic Baby Potatoes

Cooking Time: 10 minutes

Servings: 2

Ingredients:

8-ounces boiled baby potatoes

½ teaspoon sesame seeds

Red chili powder to taste

Salt and pepper to taste

½ teaspoon garlic paste

¼ teaspoon coriander seeds, dry roasted

¼ teaspoon cumin seeds, dry roasted

½ cup fresh cream

Directions:

Grind the coriander and cumin seeds to form a powder. Toss all the ingredients in a baking dish except the cream. Preheat your air fryer for 5-minutes at 360°Fahrenheit. Cook potatoes for 5-minutes. Mix in cream and air fry for an additional 5-minutes. Garnish with sesame seeds.

Mixed Cheese Corn Mash

Cooking Time: 20 minutes

Servings: 8

Ingredients:

½ cup pork rinds, chopped into small pieces

1 tablespoon butter

1 ½ cups corn kernels

¾ cup yellow onion, diced

½ cup red bell pepper, diced

¼ cup celery, diced

2 teaspoons garlic, minced

1 cup Monterey Jack cheese, grated

2 tablespoons parmesan cheese, grated

3 cups Day-old bread, cubed

¼ cup white pepper

1 ½ cups milk

½ cup heavy cream

3 eggs

Seasoning:

1 tablespoon onion powder

1 tablespoon parsley, dried

1 tablespoon thyme, dried

1 tablespoon paprika

Directions:

Use butter to grease a casserole dish. Cook the corn in a pan until it becomes caramelized for about 10-minutes. Add the onion, bell pepper, celery and cook for another 5-minutes. Mix in the thyme and garlic and remove from heat. Stir in eggs, milk, cream and whisk to combine. Add Monterey Jack cheese, bread, and cayenne pepper. Transfer mixture to casserole dish and place in air fryer basket. Cook for 30-minutes at 320°Fahrenheit. Sprinkle the top with parmesan cheese and pork rinds and cook for an additional 30-minutes.

Garlic & Ginger Snow Peas

Cooking Time: 8 minutes

Servings: 4

Ingredients:

2 cups snow peas, trimmed

1 teaspoon olive oil

1 teaspoon pepper

1 teaspoon sea salt

1 tablespoon rice vinegar

1 tablespoon tamari sauce

2 cloves garlic, minced

3-inches of ginger root, minced

Directions:

Wash the snow peas with cold running water, then trim. Clean ginger and garlic with water, then slice them into small pieces. Set them aside. In a large bowl, add a tablespoon tamari sauce, a tablespoon rice vinegar, salt, pepper, and olive oil. Mix in the minced ginger and garlic. Add trimmed snow peas and toss to combine. Soak the peas in the marinade for about an hour before air frying them. Preheat your air fryer to 380°Fahrenheit for 2-minutes. Transfer the marinated peas in a pan into air fryer and cook for 4-minutes. Toss snow peas and cook for an additional 4-minutes.

Air Fried Cabbage & Mushroom Tofu

Cooking Time: 18 minutes

Servings: 3

Ingredients:

2 teaspoons lemon zest

Salt and pepper to taste

1 tablespoon hoisin sauce

1 ½ cups tofu, cubed

1 ½ cups cabbage, shredded

1 cup mushrooms, sliced

2 tablespoons spring onions, chopped

2 teaspoons sesame oil

1 tablespoon vegan oyster sauce

Directions:

Wash the mushrooms and cabbage with water. Shred the cabbage and set aside. Cut the mushrooms thinly. Rinse and drain the tofu. Cut the tofu into small cubes. Prepare a mixing bowl, adding vegan oyster sauce, hoisin sauce, 1 teaspoon sesame oil. Add the sliced mushrooms and cabbage into the bowl and toss to combine. Let mix stand for an hour. In another bowl, combine cubed tofu and a teaspoon sesame oil. Use salt to season and allow to marinate for 30-minutes. Preheat your air fryer to 360°Fahrenehit for 2-minutes. Cook the cubed tofu for 10-minutes. Shake the air fryer basket a couple of times during the cook time. Once cooked set tofu aside. Now, cook the bowl of vegetables in air fryer basket. Cook veggies for 8-minutes. Add to a bowl with tofu and toss to combine well. Garnish with sesame seeds and chopped spring onions.

Stuffed Sweet Potato with Spinach

Cooking Time: 37 minutes

Servings: 4

Ingredients:

1 teaspoon olive oil

1 teaspoon lemon zest

4 large sweet potatoes

1 cup water spinach, steamed, chopped

1 tablespoon tamari sauce

Salt and pepper to taste

3 cloves garlic, minced

1 teaspoon cumin powder

1 teaspoon hoisin sauce

1 tablespoon lemon juice

Directions:

Wash sweet potatoes a cup of water spinach. Add your spinach in a steamer and steam for 2-minutes. In a bowl, combine a tablespoon of tamari sauce, lemon juice, hoisin sauce, minced garlic, cumin powder. Add steamed water spinach and season with salt and pepper. Set aside. Preheat your air fryer to 390°Fahrenheit for 5-minutes. Place sweet potatoes in a pan. Drizzle with lemon zest and olive oil. Place into air fryer and cook for 30-minutes. Once cooked slightly open potatoes and add the spinach mixture to them. Cook for another 5-minutes and serve warm.

Nutrition: Calories: 114, Total Fat: 0.07g, Carbs: 26.76g, Protein: 2.09g

Black Beans & Cauliflower Burgers

Cooking Time: 15 minutes

Servings: 4

Ingredients:

3 cloves garlic, minced

1 tablespoon basil leaves, minced

1 teaspoon olive oil

1 teaspoon chili sauce

1 tablespoon vegan oyster sauce

¾ cup vegan mayonnaise

4 large tomatoes, sliced

2 tablespoons potato starch

1 tablespoon flaxseed mixed with 3 tablespoons water

1 cup black beans

1 large head cauliflower, cut into florets

1 tablespoon rice vinegar

1 large avocado, mashed

Directions:

Prepare all ingredients by washing all the veggies. Cut the cauliflower, then soak it in a pot of warm water for a couple of minutes. Soak black beans in a pot of warm water with cauliflower. Rinse them with cold water, then pat dry. Check they are dry before you put them into a food processor. Add vegan oyster sauce, rice vinegar, chili sauce, and olive oil into food processor and season with salt and pepper. Add basil leaves and garlic. Now, blend until the mixture becomes rice-like in its consistency. Transfer the mixture to a bowl and set aside. Clean the food processor, then add flax seed and 3 tablespoons of water and blend mixture until it becomes fluffy. Transfer this mixture to the bowl with cauliflower mixture, add potato starch and toss to blend ingredients.

Shape burger mixture into big balls and flatten on a baking sheet to make burger patties. Now, preheat your air fryer to 360°Fahrenheit for 2-minutes. Now place enough burger patties in the air-fryer basket. Cook for 15-minutes. Make sure to flip the patties halfway through the cook time. Prepare the tomatoes and cut avocado into halves and remove the pit. Scoop the avocado flesh and mash in a bowl with a fork. Use the veggie burgers as buns. Start with one veggie burger at bottom, followed by mashed avocado, then a slice of tomato. Spread some vegan mayonnaise on top of tomato and cover with another veggie burger. Serve warm.

Nutrition: Calories: 124, Total Fat: 4.41g, Carbs: 9.99g, Protein: 10.99g

Pomelo Herb Salad with Air-Fried Brussels Sprouts

Cooking Time: 20 minutes

Servings: 5

Ingredients:

1 teaspoon olive oil

Salt and pepper to taste

1 large pomelo, peeled

2 cups Brussels sprouts, cut into halves

1 tablespoon basil leaves, chopped

1 tablespoon parsley, chopped

1 tablespoon vegan oyster sauce

2 tablespoons rice vinegar

1 tablespoon cilantro leaves, chopped

Directions:

Wash pomelo, brussels sprouts, basil, cilantro leaves. Pat dry. Peel the outer and inner skin from pomelo, leaving the pulp. Cut pulp into small bite-size pieces. Set aside. Chop parsley, basil, and brussels sprouts for later use. In a bowl, combine pomelo, basil, parsley. Add rice vinegar and sprinkle with pepper. Mix all ingredients well. In another mixing bowl, combine brussels sprouts, thyme powder, vegan oyster sauce, toss and allow to soak for 30-minutes. Preheat your air fryer to 360°Fahrenheit. Spray a teaspoon of olive oil over brussels sprouts in air fryer, then cook them for 20-minutes. Once cooked at the brussels sprouts to bowl with pomelo herb salad and toss to blend ingredients. Serve right away!

Nutrition: Calories: 46, Total Fat: 0.54g, Carbs: 9.2g, Protein: 3.48g

Spinach & Sweet Potato Curry Soup

Cooking Time: 16 minutes

Servings: 4

Ingredients:

1 cup water

3 garlic cloves, minced

1 bunch baby spinach, chopped

1 tablespoon liquid stevia

2 tablespoons coriander leaves, chopped

1 tablespoon vegan fish sauce

1 tablespoon rice vinegar

1 teaspoon lemon zest

Slices of lemon

1 large onion, sliced

1 tablespoon curry paste

1 cup rice noodles

1 cooked sweet potato, peeled and diced

Directions:

Wash veggies and pat dry. Mince the onion and garlic. Chop the baby spinach, sweet potato and coriander leaves. Set them aside. Add the noodles in a pot of boiling water, boil for 3-minutes then drain noodles. Save for later use. Preheat your air fryer to 380°Fahrenheit. Add minced garlic and onion to pan. Add sweet potato to pan. Pour in a cup of water, red curry paste, vegan fish sauce, stevia and lemon zest. Add chopped spinach and coriander. Now, season pan with salt and pepper. Place pan into air fryer and cook for 3-minutes. Add the cooked rice noodles and cook for another 5-minutes. Serve warm.

Nutrition: Calories: 214, Total Fat: 7.2g, Carbs: 26.3g, Protein: 4.2g

Jackfruit Air-Fryer Fries

Cooking Time: 20 minutes

Servings: 4

Ingredients:

1 cup Jackfruit, seeded

1 teaspoon olive oil

1 teaspoon turmeric

1 teaspoon liquid stevia

2 teaspoons sugar-free syrup

1 teaspoon salt

Directions:

In a mixing bowl, add syrup, olive oil, stevia, turmeric, and salt. Add mixture to strips of jackfruit. Toss ingredients and allow to stand for 30-minutes. Preheat your air fryer to 370°Fahrenheit for 2-minutes. Place the jackfruit into air fryer and cook for 20-minutes. Shake basket a few times through the cook time.

Nutrition: Calories: 155, Total Fat: 0.5g, Carbs: 39.2g, Protein: 2.43g

Sweet & Sour Air-Fried Yam

Cooking Time: 20 minutes

Servings: 4

Ingredients:

1 teaspoon olive oil

2 tablespoons chives, minced

Salt and pepper to taste

1 teaspoon lemon zest

1 tablespoon liquid stevia

1 tablespoon tamarind paste

2 cups Yam, cut into strips

Directions:

Wash the veggies and peel the skin from yams. Cut the yams into strips and put in a mixing bowl. Add stevia and tamarind paste into a bowl. Add minced chives into a bowl. Season with salt and pepper. Sprinkle with lemon zest. Marinate yams for 30-minutes. Preheat your air-fryer to 380°Fahrenheit. Add yams to the air-fryer basket and spray teaspoon of olive oil on jicama. Cook for 20-minutes until crispy. Shake the basket a few times during cook time. Serve warm.

Nutrition: Calories: 49, Total Fat: 0.12g, Carbs: 11.47g, Proteins: 0.94g

Avocado Bites

Preparation time: 5 minutes

Cooking time: 10 minutes

Servings: 4

Ingredients:

2 teaspoons garlic powder

2 avocados, peeled, pitted and sliced

Salt and black pepper to the taste

1 tablespoon balsamic vinegar

A drizzle of olive oil

1 teaspoon coriander, ground

Directions:

In your air fryer's basket, combine the avocado pieces with garlic powder and the other ingredients, toss and cook at 350 degrees F for 10 minutes.

Divide into bowls and serve as a snack.

Nutrition: calories 210, fat 19.6, fiber 6.9, carbs 9.7, protein 2.2

Radish Chips

Preparation time: 5 minutes

Cooking time: 12 minutes

Servings: 4

Ingredients:

1 pound radishes, thinly sliced

1 tablespoon lime juice

1 tablespoon avocado oil

A pinch of salt and black pepper

1 teaspoon red pepper flakes, crushed

Directions:

In your air fryer's basket, combine the radish chips with the lime juice and the other ingredients, toss and cook at 380 degrees F for 12 minutes.

 Transfer to bowls and serve as a snack.

Nutrition: calories 24, fat 0.6, fiber 2.1, carbs 4.3, protein 0.9

Apple Dip

Preparation time: 5 minutes

Cooking time: 12 minutes

Servings: 4

Ingredients:

4 big apples, cored, peeled and cubed

2 teaspoons lemon juice

½ cup apple juice

1 teaspoon nutmeg, ground

Directions:

In a blender, combine the apples with the lemon juice and the other ingredients, pulse well and divide into 4 ramekins.

Put the ramekins in the air fryer's basket and cook everything at 340 degrees F for 12 minutes.

Serve as a party dip.

Nutrition: calories 134, fat 34.6, fiber 5.6, carbs 34.6, protein 0.7

Zucchini Spread

Preparation time: 10 minutes

Cooking time: 15 minutes

Servings: 6

Ingredients:

1 pound zucchinis, grated

1 cup heavy cream

1 tablespoon avocado oil

1 tablespoon lime juice

1 teaspoon dill, chopped

Salt and black pepper to the taste

2 garlic cloves, minced

Directions:

In a bowl, combine the zucchinis with the cream and the other ingredients, whisk well and pour into 6 ramekins.

Place the ramekins in your air fryer's basket, cook at 375 degrees F for 15 minutes and serve as an appetizer.

Nutrition: calories 86, fat 7.9, fiber 1, carbs 3.6, protein 1.4

Basil Dip

Preparation time: 10 minutes

Cooking time: 15 minutes

Servings: 4

Ingredients:

1 cup basil leaves

1 cup heavy cream

1 avocado, peeled, pitted and cubed

1 tablespoon olive oil

4 scallions, chopped

Salt and black pepper to the taste

1 garlic clove, minced

Directions:

In a blender, combine the basil with the cream and the other ingredients, pulse well and divide into 4 ramekins

Put the ramekins in the fryer's basket and cook at 350 degrees F for 15 minutes.

Serve as a party dip.

Nutrition: calories 243, fat 24.5, fiber 3.9, carbs 6.7, protein 2.1

Tomato Dip

Preparation time: 10 minutes

Cooking time: 20 minutes

Servings: 4

Ingredients:

1 pound tomatoes

Salt and black pepper to the taste

2 tablespoons avocado oil

2 tablespoons balsamic vinegar

1 tablespoon basil, chopped

1 cup heavy cream

Directions:

In your air fryer's basket, combine the tomatoes with the oil and the other ingredients except the cream, toss and cook at 220 degrees F for 20 minutes.

Peel and transfer the tomatoes to a blender, add the cream, pulse, divide into bowls and serve.

Nutrition: calories 135, fat 12.2, fiber 1.7, carbs 5.7, protein 1.7

Paprika Carrot Dip

Preparation time: 10 minutes

Cooking time: 20 minutes

Servings: 4

Ingredients:

1 pound carrots, peeled and sliced

1 teaspoon sweet paprika

1 cup tomato passata

1 teaspoon rosemary, dried

Salt and black pepper to the taste

½ teaspoon turmeric powder

1 teaspoon olive oil

Directions:

In your air fryer's pan, combine the carrots with the paprika and the other ingredients, whisk and cook at 370 degrees F for 20 minutes

Transfer the mix to a blender, pulse, divide into bowls and serve as a snack.

Nutrition: calories 161, fat 1, fiber 2, carbs 5, protein 3

Chives Olives Bowls

Preparation time: 10 minutes

Cooking time: 12 minutes

Servings: 4

Ingredients:

1 cup black olives, pitted

1 cup kalamata olives, pitted

1 cup green olives, pitted

1 tablespoon lime juice

1 teaspoon rosemary, dried

A drizzle of olive oil

Salt and black pepper to the taste

1 tablespoon chives, chopped

Directions:

In your air fryer's basket, combine the olives with the lime juice and the other ingredients, toss and cook at 350 degrees F for 12 minutes.

Divide into bowls and serve as a snack..

Nutrition: calories 100, fat 1, fiber 2, carbs 4, protein 1

Lentils Spread

Preparation time: 10 minutes

Cooking time: 12 minutes

Servings: 4

Ingredients:

15 ounces canned lentils, drained

½ teaspoon basil, dried

2 tablespoons olive oil

1 cup heavy cream

1 teaspoon sweet paprika

Salt and black pepper to the taste

Directions:

In your air fryer's pan, combine the lentils with the basil and the other ingredients, whisk and cook at 380 degrees F for 12 minutes.

Blend using an immersion blender, divide into bowls and serve.

Nutrition: calories 151, fat 1, fiber 6, carbs 10, protein 6

Roasted Chickpeas

Preparation time: 5 minutes

Cooking time: 12 minutes

Servings: 4

Ingredients:

2 cups canned chickpeas, drained and rinsed

2 and ½ tablespoons butter, melted

1 teaspoon chili powder

1 teaspoon coriander, ground

A pinch of salt and black pepper

Directions:

In your air fryer, combine the chickpeas with the butter and the other ingredients, toss and cook at 400 degrees F for 12 minutes.

Serve as a snack.

Nutrition: calories 70, fat 2, fiber 2, carbs 7, protein 3

Shrimp and Mango Platter

Preparation time: 5 minutes

Cooking time: 8 minutes

Servings: 4

Ingredients:

1 pound shrimp, deveined and peeled

2 mangoes, peeled and roughly cubed

1 cup baby spinach

2 tablespoons olive oil

1 tablespoon balsamic vinegar

Salt and black pepper to the taste

Directions:

In your air fryer, combine the shrimp with the mango and the other ingredients, toss and cook at 370 degrees F for 8 minutes

Arrange the whole mix on a platter and serve as an appetizer.

Nutrition: calories 150, fat 4, fiber 3, carbs 13, protein 4

Fish Strips

Preparation time: 10 minutes

Cooking time: 16 minutes

Servings: 4

Ingredients:

¾ cup almond flour

1 pound cod fillets, boneless, skinless and cut into strips

1 egg, whisked

1 teaspoon rosemary, dried

1 teaspoon turmeric powder

Salt and black pepper to the taste

Cooking spray

Directions:

In a bowl, mix the flour with salt and pepper.

Put the egg in another bowl.

Dredge the fish in flour and egg, place the strips in your lined air fryer's basket, grease them with cooking spray, cook at 400 degrees F for 16 minutes, flipping them halfway and serve as an appetizer.

Nutrition: calories 181, fat 4, fiber 7, carbs 15, protein 18

Olive and Beef Balls

Preparation time: 10 minutes

Cooking time: 14 minutes

Servings: 8

Ingredients:

1 pound beef meat, minced

1 cup kalamata olives, pitted and chopped

1 tablespoon chives, chopped

Salt and black pepper to the taste

1 tablespoon bread crumbs

1 tablespoon oregano, chopped

Cooking spray

Directions:

In a bowl, mix the beef with the olives and the other ingredients except the cooking spray, shape medium balls out of this mix, and place them in your air fryer's basket.

Grease them with the cooking spray, cook at 400 degrees F for 14 minutes flipping them halfway, arrange them on a platter and serve as an appetizer.

Nutrition: calories 194, fat 9, fiber 2, carbs 11, protein 15

Cheesy Peppers Spread

Preparation time: 5 minutes

Cooking time: 14 minutes

Servings: 6

Ingredients:

10 ounces roasted peppers, chopped

1 tablespoon olive oil

1 cup heavy cream

Salt and black pepper to the taste

A pinch of cayenne pepper

2 tablespoons oregano, chopped

Directions:

In your air fryer's pan, combine the peppers with the oil, cream and the other ingredients, stir and cook at 370 degrees F for 14 minutes.

Blend using an immersion blender, divide into bowls and serve as a party spread.

Nutrition: calories 150, fat 1, fiber 2, carbs 7, protein 5

Avocado Tomato Salsa

Preparation time: 4 minutes

Cooking time: 8 minutes

Servings: 6

Ingredients:

½ pound cherry tomatoes, halved

1 avocado, peeled, pitted and cubed

1 tablespoon balsamic vinegar

½ cup black olives, pitted and sliced

Salt and black pepper to the taste

2 tablespoons basil, chopped

1 tablespoons shallots, chopped

Directions:

In your air fryer's pan, combine the tomatoes with the avocado, vinegar and the other ingredients, toss and cook at 360 degrees F for 8 minutes.

Divide into bowls and serve as a snack.

Nutrition: calories 140, fat 1, fiber 4, carbs 8, protein 3

Shrimp Dip

Preparation time: 5 minutes

Cooking time: 8 minutes

Servings: 6

Ingredients:

2 tablespoons olive oil

1 pound shrimp, peeled, deveined and chopped

1 tablespoons mint, chopped

1 cup heavy cream

1 teaspoon turmeric powder

1 teaspoon chili powder

Directions:

In your air fryer's pan, mix the shrimp with the mint, oil and the other ingredients, stir, and cook at 380 degrees F for 8 minutes.

Divide into bowls and serve as a party dip.

Nutrition: calories 194, fat 4, fiber 2, carbs 12, protein 7

Mozzarella Spread

Preparation time: 5 minutes

Cooking time: 10 minutes

Servings: 6

Ingredients:

1 cup heavy cream

Salt and black pepper to the taste

1 and ½ cups mozzarella, shredded

1 tablespoon cilantro, chopped

1 tablespoon chives, chopped

1 tablespoon Italian seasoning

Directions:

In a bowl, mix the heavy cream with the mozzarella and the other ingredients, stir well and divide into 6 ramekins.

Put the ramekins in the air fryer's basket and cook at 390 degrees F for 10 minutes.

Serve the spread warm.

Nutrition: calories 200, fat 5, fiber 3, carbs 13, protein 4

Kale Spread

Preparation time: 10 minutes

Cooking time: 20 minutes

Servings: 6

Ingredients:

4 bunches kale, torn

1 cup heavy cream

4 garlic cloves, minced

2 tablespoons avocado oil

A pinch of salt and black pepper

1 teaspoon coriander, ground

Directions:

In a blender, combine the kale with the cream and the other ingredients, pulse well, transfer air fryer's pan, cook at 380 degrees F for 20 minutes, divide into bowls and serve cold as a party spread.

Nutrition: calories 153, fat 1, fiber 2, carbs 11, protein 5

Air Fried Chicken Thighs

Cooking Time: 12 minutes

Servings: 2

Ingredients:

2 boneless chicken thighs

Salt and pepper to taste

1 teaspoon rosemary, dried

1 tablespoon Worcestershire sauce

1 tablespoon oyster sauce

1 teaspoon liquid stevia

2 garlic cloves, minced

Directions:

Add ingredients to a bowl and combine well. Place the marinated chicken in the fridge for an hour. Preheat your air fryer to 180°Fahrenheit for 3-minutes. Add marinated chicken to air fryer grill pan and cook for 12-minutes. Serve hot!

Nutrition: Calories: 270, Total Fat: 17g, Carbs: 7g, Protein: 20g

Chicken Cheese Fillet

Cooking Time: 15 minutes

Servings: 4

Ingredients:

2 large chicken fillets

4 Gouda cheese slices

 4 ham slices

Salt and Pepper to taste

1 tablespoon of chives, chopped

Directions:

Preheat your air fryer to 180°Fahrenheit. Cut chicken fillet into four pieces. Make a slit horizontally to the edge. Open the fillet and season with salt and pepper. Cover each piece with chives and cheese slice. Close fillet and wrap in a ham slice. Place wrap chicken fillet into air fryer basket and cook for 15-minutes. Serve hot!

Nutrition: Calories: 386, Total Fat: 21g, Carbs: 14.3g, Protein: 30g

Roasted Pepper Salad

Cooking Time: 10 minutes

Servings: 4

Ingredients:

1 lettuce cut into broad strips

1 red bell pepper

1 tablespoon lemon juice

3 tablespoons of rocket leaves

Black pepper to taste

2 tablespoons olive oil

3 tablespoons plain yogurt

Directions:

Preheat your air fryer to 200°Fahrenheit. Place the bell pepper in air fryer basket and roast for 10-minutes. Add pepper to a bowl, cover with a lid and set aside for 10-minutes. Cut bell pepper into four parts and remove the seeds and skin. Chop the bell pepper into strips. Add lemon juice, yogurt, and oil in a bowl. Season with black pepper. Add lettuce and rocket leaves and toss. Garnish the salad with red bell pepper strips. Serve and enjoy!

Nutrition: Calories: 91, Total Fat: 7g, Carbs: 3g, Protein: 2g

Pineapple Pizza

Cooking Time: 10 minutes

Servings: 3

Ingredients:

1 large whole wheat tortilla

¼ cup tomato pizza sauce

¼ cup pineapple tidbits

¼ cup mozzarella cheese, grated

¼ cup ham slice

Directions:

Preheat your air fryer to 300°Fahrenehit. Place the tortilla on a baking sheet then spread pizza sauce over tortilla. Arrange ham slice, cheese, pineapple over the tortilla. Place the pizza in the air fryer basket and cook for 10-minutes. Serve hot。

Nutrition: Calories: 80, Total Fat: 2g, Carbs: 12g, Protein: 4g

Air Fryer Tortilla Pizza

Cooking Time: 7 minutes

Servings: 6

Ingredients:

1 large whole wheat tortilla

1 tablespoon black olives

Salt and pepper to taste

4 tablespoons tomato sauce

8 pepperoni slices

3 tablespoons of sweet corn

1 medium, tomato, chopped

½ cup mozzarella cheese, grated

Directions:

Preheat your air fryer to 325°Fahrenheit. Spread tomato sauce over tortilla. Add pepperoni slices, olives, corn, tomato, and cheese on top of the tortilla. Season with salt and pepper. Place pizza in air fryer basket and cook for 7-minutes. Serve and enjoy!

Nutrition: Calories: 110, Total Fat: 5g, Carbs: 10g, Protein: 4g

Air Fried Pork Apple Balls

Cooking Time: 15 minutes

Servings: 8

Ingredients:

2 cups pork, minced

6 basil leaves, chopped

2 tablespoons cheddar cheese, grated

4 garlic cloves, minced

½ cup apple, peeled, cored, chopped

1 large white onion, diced

Salt and pepper to taste

2 teaspoons Dijon Mustard

1 teaspoon liquid Stevia

Directions:

Add pork minced in a bowl then add diced onion and apple into a bowl and mix well. Add the stevia, mustard, garlic, cheese, basil, salt and pepper and combine well. Make small round balls from the mixture and place them into air fryer basket. Cook at 350°Fahrenheit for 15-minutes. Serve and enjoy!

Stuffed Garlic Chicken

Cooking Time: 15 minutes

Servings: 2

Ingredients:

¼ cup of tomatoes, sliced

½ tablespoon garlic, minced

2 basil leaves

Salsa for serving

1 prosciutto slice

2 teaspoons parmesan cheese, freshly grated

2 boneless chicken breasts

Pepper and salt to taste

Directions:

Cut the side of the chicken breast to make a pocket. Stuff each pocket with tomato slices, garlic, grated cheese and basil leaves. Cut a slice of prosciutto in half to form 2 equal size pieces. Season chicken with salt and pepper and wrap each with a slice of prosciutto. Preheat your air fryer to 325°Fahrenheit. Place the stuffed chicken breasts into air fryer basket and cook for 15-minutes. Serve chicken breasts with salsa.

Rosemary Citrus Chicken

Cooking Time: 15 minutes

Servings: 2

Ingredients:

1 lb. chicken thighs

1/2 teaspoon rosemary, fresh, chopped

1/8 teaspoon thyme, dried

½ cup tangerine juice

2 tablespoons white wine

1 teaspoon garlic, minced

Salt and pepper to taste

2 tablespoons lemon juice

Directions:

Place the chicken thighs in a mixing bowl. In another bowl, mix tangerine juice, garlic, white wine, lemon juice, rosemary, pepper, salt, and thyme. Pour the mixture over chicken thighs and place in the fridge for 20-minutes. Preheat your air fryer to 350°Fahrenheit and place your marinated chicken in air fryer basket and cook for 15-minutes. Serve hot and enjoy!

Nutrition: Calories: 473, Total Fat: 17g, Carbs: 7g, Protein: 66g

Air Fried Garlic Popcorn Chicken

Cooking Time: 15 minutes

Servings: 6

Ingredients:

1 lb. chicken breasts, skinless,

boneless, cut into bite-size chunks

¼ teaspoon garlic powder

Salt and pepper to taste

¼ teaspoon paprika

¼ cup of buttermilk

1 tablespoon olive oil

½ cup gluten-free flour

2 cups corn flakes

2 tablespoons parmesan cheese, grated

Directions:

Preheat your air fryer to 350°Fahrenheit. In a bowl, mix garlic, chicken, pepper, and salt. Add cornflakes, parmesan cheese, pepper, paprika, and salt into food processor and process mix until it forms a crumble. In a shallow dish add flour. In another bowl add the crumbled cornflake mixture. Add chicken pieces to the flour and coat well. Drizzle buttermilk over the coated chicken pieces and mix well. Coat chicken pieces with cornflakes mixture. Add coated chicken pieces onto a baking sheet and place in the air fryer basket. Drizzle the olive oil over popcorn chicken. Bake in preheated air fryer for 15-minutes. Serve warm!

Nutrition: Calories: 235, Total Fat: 8g, Carbs: 14g, Protein: 23g

Macaroni Cheese Toast

Cooking Time: 5 minutes

Servings: 2

Ingredients:

1 egg, beaten

4 tablespoons cheddar cheese, grated

Salt and pepper to taste

½ cup macaroni and cheese

4 bread slices

Directions:

Spread the cheese and macaroni and cheese over the two bread slices. Place the other bread slices on top of cheese and cut diagonally. In a bowl, beat egg and season with salt and pepper. Brush the egg mixture onto the bread. Place the bread into air fryer and cook at 300°Fahrenehit for 5-minutes.

Nutrition: Calories: 250, Total Fat: 16g, Carbs: 9g, Protein: 14g

Cheese Burger Patties

Cooking Time: 15 minutes

Servings: 6

Ingredients:

1 lb. ground beef

6 cheddar cheese slices

Pepper and salt to taste

Directions:

Preheat your air fryer to 390°Fahrenheit. Season beef with salt and pepper. Make six round shaped patties from the mixture and place them into air fryer basket. Air fry the patties for 10-minutes. Open the air fryer basket and place cheese slices on top of patties and place into air fryer with an additional cook time of 1-minute.

Nutrition: Calories: 253, Total Fat: 14g, Carbs: 0.4g, Protein: 29g

Grilled Cheese Corn

Cooking Time: 15 minutes

Servings: 2

Ingredients:

2 whole corn on the cob, peel husks and discard silk

1 teaspoon olive oil

2 teaspoons paprika

½ cup feta cheese, grated

Directions:

Rub the olive oil over corn then sprinkle with paprika and rub all over the corn. Preheat your air fryer to 300°Fahrenheit. Place the seasoned corn on the grill for 15-minutes. Place corn on a serving dish then sprinkle with grated cheese over corn. Serve and enjoy!

Nutrition: Calories: 150, Total Fat: 10g, Carbs: 7g, Protein: 7g

Eggplant Fries

Cooking Time: 20 minutes

Servings: 4

Ingredients:

1 eggplant, cut into 3-inch pieces

¼ cup of water

1 tablespoon of olive oil

4 tablespoons cornstarch

Sea salt to taste

Directions:

Preheat your air fryer to 390°Fahrenheit. In a bowl, combine eggplant, water, oil, and cornstarch. Place the eggplant fries in air fryer basket, and air fry them for 20-minutes. Serve warm and enjoy!

Air Fried Pita Bread Pizza

Cooking Time: 6 minutes

Servings: 3

Ingredients:

1 large pita bread

1 teaspoon olive oil

7 pepperoni slices

¼ cup of sausage

½ teaspoon garlic, minced

1 tablespoon pizza sauce

¼ cup mozzarella cheese, shredded

1 small onion, finely diced

Directions:

Spread the pizza sauce over the pita bread evenly. Arrange pepperoni, onion, and sausage over pita bread. Sprinkle the top with garlic and cheese. Drizzle the pizza with olive oil then place in air basket. Place on top of trivet and air fry at 350°Fahrenheit for 6-minutes. Serve and enjoy!

Eggplant fries

Preparation time: 5 minutes

Cooking time: 15 minutes

Servings: 2 to 4 people

Ingredients:

2 large eggs

½ cup of grated Parmesan cheese

½ cup of toasted wheat germ

1 tsp. of Italian seasoning

¾ tsp. of garlic salt

1 medium eggplant (about 1-1/4 pounds

Cooking spray

1 cup meatless pasta sauce, warmed

Cooking Directions:

Preheat air fryer to 400°F, In a shallow bowl, whisk eggs. In another shallow bowl, mix cheese, wheat germ and seasonings.

Cut eggplant lengthwise into ½ -in.-thick slices. Cut slices lengthwise into ½ -in. strips. Dip eggplant in eggs, then coat with cheese mixture.

Spritz eggplant and air fryer basket with cooking spray. Working in batches if needed, place eggplant in a single layer in air fryer basket.

Cook until golden brown, for about 10 minutes. Turn eggplant; spritz with additional cooking spray.

Continue cooking until golden brown, for about 5 minutes. Serve immediately with pasta dipping sauce.

Raspberry Balsamic Smoked Pork Chops

Preparation time: 15 minutes

Cooking time: 15 minutes

Servings: 4 to 6 people

Ingredients:

2 large eggs

¼ cup of milk

1 cup of panko (Japanese bread crumbs

1 cup of finely chopped pecans

4 smoked bone-in pork chops (7-1/2 ounces each

1/4 cup of all-purpose flour

1/3 cup of balsamic vinegar

2 tbsp. of brown sugar

2 tbsp. of seedless raspberry jam

1 tbsp. of thawed frozen orange juice concentrate

Directions:

Preheat air fryer to 400°F and spritz air fryer basket with cooking spray. In a shallow bowl, whisk together eggs and milk.

In another shallow bowl, toss bread crumbs with pecans. Coat pork chops with flour and shake off excess.

Dip in egg mixture, then in crumb mixture, patting to help adhere. Working in batches as needed, place chops in single layer in air fryer basket.

Spritz with cooking spray. Cook until golden brown, for about 15 minutes, turning halfway through cooking and spritzing with additional cooking spray.

Remove and keep warm. Repeat with remaining chops. Meanwhile, place remaining ingredients in a small saucepan; bring to a boil.

Cook and stir until slightly thickened, for about 8 minutes. Serve with chops.

Pickles

Preparation time: 20 minutes

Cook time: 15 minutes

Servings: 8 to 12 people

Ingredients:

32 dill pickle slices

½ cup of all-purpose flour

½ tsp. of salt

3 large eggs, lightly beaten

2 tbsp. of dill pickle juice

½ tsp. of cayenne pepper

1/2 tsp. of garlic powder

2 cups of panko (Japanese bread crumbs

2 tbsp. of snipped fresh dill

Cooking spray

Ranch salad dressing, optional

Cooking Directions:

Preheat air fryer to 425°F and let pickles stand on a paper towel until liquid is almost absorbed, for about 15 minutes.

Meanwhile, in a shallow bowl, combine flour and salt. In another shallow bowl, whisk eggs, pickle juice, cayenne and garlic powder.

Combine panko and dill in a third shallow bowl. Dip pickles in flour mixture to coat both sides, shake off excess.

Dip in egg mixture, then in crumb mixture, patting to help coating adhere. Spritz pickles and fryer basket with cooking spray.

Working in batches if needed, place pickles in a single layer in basket and cook until golden brown and crispy, for about 10 minutes.

Turn pickles; spritz with additional cooking spray. Continue cooking until golden brown and crispy, for about 10 minutes.

Serve immediately. If desired, serve with ranch dressing.

Garlic-Rosemary Brussels Sprouts

Preparation time: 5 minutes

Cooking time: 30 minutes

Servings: 2 to 4 people

Ingredients:

3 tbsp. of olive oil

2 garlic cloves, minced

½ tsp. of salt

¼ tsp. of pepper

1 lb. of Brussels sprouts, trimmed and halved

1/2 cup of panko (Japanese bread crumbs

1 ½ tsp. of minced fresh rosemary

Cooking Directions:

Preheat air fryer to 350°F and place first 4 ingredients in a small microwave-safe bowl; microwave on high for about 30 seconds.

Toss Brussels sprouts with 2 tablespoons oil mixture. Place all the Brussels sprouts in fryer basket and cook for about 5 minutes.

Stir sprouts. Continue to air-fry until sprouts are lightly browned and near desired tenderness, for about 8 minutes longer, stirring halfway through cooking time.

Toss bread crumbs with rosemary and remaining oil mixture; sprinkle over sprouts.

Continue cooking until crumbs are browned and sprouts are tender, for about 5 minutes. Serve immediately and Enjoy!

Chocolate Chip Oatmeal

Preparation time: 10 minutes

Cooking time: 20 minutes

Servings: 4 to 6 people

Ingredients:

1 cup of butter, softened

¾ cup of sugar

¾ cup of packed brown sugar

2 large eggs

1 tsp. of vanilla extract

3 cups of quick-cooking oats

1 ½ cups of all-purpose flour

1 package (3.4 ounces of instant vanilla pudding mix

1 tsp. of baking soda

1 tsp. of salt

2 cups (12 ounces of semisweet chocolate chips

1 cup of chopped nuts

Cooking Directions:

Preheat fryer to 350°F and line fryer basket with foil. In a large bowl, cream butter and sugars until light and fluffy.

Beat in eggs and vanilla. Combine the oats, flour, dry pudding mix, baking soda and salt; gradually add to creamed mixture and mix well.

Stir in chocolate chips and nuts. Form into balls using 1 tablespoon of dough; flatten slightly.

Place shaped dough 2 in. apart onto foil-lined fryer basket. Air- fry until lightly browned, for about 10 minutes.

Remove to wire racks. Repeat with remaining dough.

Reuben Calzones

Preparation time: 15 minutes

Cooking time: 10 minutes

Servings: 2 to 4 people

Ingredients:

1 tube (13.8 ounces of refrigerated pizza crust

4 slices of Swiss cheese

1 cup of sauerkraut, rinsed and well drained

1/2 lb. of sliced cooked corned beef

Thousand Island salad dressing

Cooking Directions:

Preheat air fryer to 400F° and spritz air fryer basket with cooking spray. On a lightly floured surface, unroll pizza crust dough and pat into a 12-in. square.

Cut into 4 squares. Layer one slice of the cheese and a fourth of the sauerkraut and corned beef diagonally over half of each square to within ½ in. of edges.

Fold 1 corner over filling to the opposite corner, forming a triangle; press edges with a fork to seal. Place 2 calzones in a single layer in greased fryer basket.

Cook until calzones are golden brown, for about 15 minutes, flipping halfway through cooking. Remove and keep warm; repeat with remaining calzones.

Serve with salad dressing.

Coconut Shrimp

Preparation time: 10 minutes

Cooking time: 15 minutes

Servings: 8 to 12 people

Cooking Ingredients:

12 wild caught XL shrimp

1/3 cup of cassava flour I like Otto's Cassava Flour

2 large eggs, beaten

1/2 cup of unsweetened shredded coconut

1 lime wedge

1 tbsp. of extra virgin olive oil for brushing the basket.

Tropical Dipping Sauce

4 tsp. of coconut amino

1 cup of pineapple juice

1 tsp. of raw honey

¼ tsp. of ginger powder

½ tsp. of tapioca starch

Directions:

Wash the shrimp and devein them. Make small slits in the belly of the shrimps, so they don't curl when cooked.

Place cassava flour on a plate, the eggs in a shallow bowl, and the shredded coconut on another plate.

Dredge shrimp in the flour, dip in the egg and roll and coat with the shredded coconut. Refrigerate for about 30 minutes. Preheat the air fryer to 360°F.

Brush the basket with extra virgin olive oil. Place 6 shrimp in the basket, in a single layer, and set the timer for 7 minutes.

Meanwhile, in a small saucepan, bring the pineapple juice to a boil and then simmer on low heat, until it's reduced to half.

Add the rest of the ingredients and stir well. Remove pan from heat and set it aside. When the timer goes off, take the shrimp out, place them on a plate, and cover.

Put the rest of the shrimp in the basket and cook for 7 minutes. When the timer goes off, squeeze some lime juice on the shrimp.

8.   Serve immediately with the tropical dipping sauce.

Air-Fried Asparagus

Preparation time: 5 minutes

Cooking time: 10 minutes

Servings: 2 to 4 people

Ingredients:

½ bunch of asparagus, with bottom 2 inches trimmed off

Avocado or Olive Oil in an oil mister or sprayer

Himalayan salt

Black pepper

Directions:

Place trimmed asparagus spears in the air-fryer basket.

Spritz spears lightly with oil, then sprinkle with salt and a tiny bit of black pepper.

Place basket inside air-fryer and bake at 400° for 10 minutes. Serve immediately and Enjoy!

Roasted Asian Broccoli

Preparation time: 10 minutes

Cooking time: 20 minutes

Servings: 2 to 4 people

Ingredients:

1 pound of broccoli, cut into florets

1 1/2 tablespoons of peanut oil

1 tablespoon of garlic, minced

Salt

2 tablespoons of reduced sodium soy sauce

2 teaspoon of honey (or agave

2 teaspoons of sriracha

1 teaspoon of rice vinegar

1/3 cup of roasted salted peanuts

Fresh lime juice (optional

Directions:

In a large bowl, toss together the broccoli, peanut oil, garlic and season with sea salt. Make sure the oil covers all the broccoli florets.

Spread the broccoli into the wire basket of your air fryer, in as single of a layer, as possible, trying to leave a little bit of space between each floret.

Cook at 4000F until golden brown and crispy, for about 15 to 20 minutes, stirring halfway.

While the broccoli and peanuts cook, mix together the honey, soy sauce, sriracha and rice vinegar in a small, microwave-safe bowl.

Once mixed, microwave the mixture for about 10 to 15 seconds until the honey is melted, and evenly incorporated.

Transfer the cooked broccoli to a bowl and add in the soy sauce mixture. Toss to coat and season to taste with a pinch more salt, if needed.

Stir in the peanuts and squeeze lime on top. Serve immediately and Enjoy!

Chicken nuggets

Preparation time: 10 minutes

Cooking time: 8 minutes

Servings: 2 to 4 people

Ingredients:

1 boneless skinless chicken breast

¼ tsp. of salt

1/8 tsp. of black pepper

½ cup of unsalted butter melted

½ cup of breadcrumbs

2 tbsp. of grated parmesan optional

Directions:

Preheat air fryer to 3900F for about 4 minutes. Trim any fat from chicken breast, Slice into 1/2-inch thick slices, then each slice into 2 to 3 nuggets.

Season chicken pieces with salt and pepper. Place melted butter in a small bowl and breadcrumbs (with Parmesan in another small bowl.

Dip each piece of chicken in butter, then breadcrumbs. Place in a single layer in the air fryer basket.

Depending on the size of your air fryer, you may need to bake in two batches or more. Set timer to 8 minutes.

When done, check if the internal temperature of chicken nuggets is at least 1650F. Remove nuggets from basket with tongs and set onto a plate to cool.

Serve immediately and Enjoy!

Churro Bites

Preparation time: 5 minutes

Cooking time: 20 minutes

Servings: 2 to 4 people

Ingredients:

1 cup of water

8 tbsp. (1 stick of unsalted butter, cut into 8 pieces

½ cup + 1 tbsp. of granulated sugar, divided

1 cup of all-purpose flour

1 tsp. of vanilla extract

3 large eggs

2 tsp. of ground cinnamon

4 oz. of finely chopped dark chocolate

¼ cup sour cream or Greek yogurt

Directions:

Bring the water, butter, and 1 tablespoon of the sugar to a simmer in a small saucepan over medium-high heat.

Add the flour and quickly stir it in with a sturdy wooden spoon. Continue to cook, stirring constantly, until the flour smells toasted and the mixture is thick, for about 3 minutes.

Transfer to a large bowl. Using the same wooden spoon, beat the flour mixture until cooled slightly but still warm, about 1 minute of constant stirring.

Stir in the vanilla. Stir in the eggs one at a time, making sure each egg is incorporated before adding the next.

Transfer the dough to a piping bag or gallon zip-top bag. Let the dough rest for 1 hour at room temperature.

Meanwhile, prepare the cinnamon sugar and chocolate sauce. Combine the cinnamon and remaining ½ cup sugar in large bowl.

Microwave the chocolate in a medium microwave-safe mixing bowl in 30-second intervals, stirring between each, until the chocolate is melted, for about 2 minutes.

8.   Add the sour cream or yogurt and whisk until smooth. Cover and set aside. Preheat the air fryer for about 10 minutes at 375°F.

Pipe the batter directly into the preheated air fryer, making 6 (3-inch pieces and piping them at least ½ -inch apart.

10. Air fry until golden-brown, for about 10 minutes. Immediately transfer the churros to the bowl of cinnamon sugar and toss to coat.

11. Repeat with air frying the remaining batter. Serve the churros warm with the dipping sauce.

Apple chips

Preparation time: 5 minutes

Cooking time: 8 minutes

Overall time:13 minutes

Servings: 2 to 4 people

Ingredients:

3 large sweet, crisp apples

¾ tsp. of ground cinnamon

A pinch of salt

Directions:

Wash the apples in warn water or apple cider vinegar thoroughly. You can either core the apples or if you are like just leave the seeds in there.

Preheat the air fryer at 3900F. Using a mandolin or sharp knife, cut the apple sideways into 1/8th inch rounds.

Mix cinnamon and salt in a bowl. Arrange apples in a single layer and sprinkle or rub some cinnamon and salt mixture.

Arrange a single layer of the above apple slices in the air fryer. Cook for about 8 minutes at 3900F, flipping sides half way through.

First batch should be ready in 8 minutes. Repeat above step for other batches. Once you are happy with the crispiness, cool the chips on a cooling rack.

Enjoy them as is or store them into an air tight container.

Baked Potatoes

Preparation time: 2 minutes

Cooking time: 40 minutes

Servings: 1 to 3 people

Ingredients:

3 russet potatoes (medium sized, scrubbed and rinsed

Cooking spray (I used avocado oil spray

½ tsp. of sea salt (use a bit less if you are using a finer salt, like table salt

½ tsp. of garlic powder

Directions:

Place your potatoes in the Air Fryer basket, and spray with cooking spray on both sides. Sprinkle sea salt and garlic on all sides, rotating the potatoes as you got.

Use your hands to rub the potatoes to make sure everything becomes evenly coated.

Cook in the Air Fryer at 4000F, for about 40 to 50 minutes, until fork tender. Serve immediately and Enjoy!

Mushroom Rice

Preparation time: 5 minutes

Cooking time: 20 minutes

Servings: 4 to 6 people

Ingredients:

16 oz. of jasmine rice uncooked

½ cup of soy sauce you can use gluten free tamari

4 tbsp. of maple syrup

4 cloves of garlic finely chopped

2 tsp. of Chinese 5 Spice

½ tsp. of ground ginger

4 tbsp. of white wine you can use rice vinegar

16 oz. of cremini mushrooms wiped clean, you can cut any huge mushrooms in half

½ cup of peas frozen

Directions:

Start your rice now so that it will be done and hot at the same time as the sauce. Mix the next 6 ingredients together and set it aside.

Place the mushrooms in the air fryer. Set it to 350F and cook for about 10 minutes. Open the air fryer, if you don't have one that stirs itself, pull out the pot and shake.

Pour the liquid mixture and peas over the top of the mushrooms. Stir and cook 5 more minutes.

Pour the mushroom/pea sauce over the pot of rice and stir. Serve immediately and Enjoy!

Air fried steak

Preparation time: 5 minutes

Cooking time: 12 minutes

Servings: 1 to 3 people

Ingredients:

2 to 12 ounces of strip steaks (1 inch thick

Salt and Pepper to taste

2 tbsp. of butter (optional

Directions:

Preheat your air fryer. Set the temperature to 4000F.

Season your steak with salt and pepper on each side. Place the steak in your air fryer basket.

Do not overlap the steaks. Set the time to 12 minutes and flip the steak at 6. Serve with vegetables or mashed cauliflower.

Hash Brown

Preparation time: 15 minutes

Cooking time: 15 minutes

Servings: 6 to 8 people

Ingredients:

4 peeled and finely grated large potatoes

2 tbsp. of corn flour

Salt to taste

Pepper powder - to taste

2 tsp. chili flakes

1 tsp. garlic powder (optional

1 tsp. of onion Powder - (optional

2 tsp. of vegetable oil

Directions:

Soak the shredded potatoes in cold water and drain the water. Repeat the step to drain excess starch from potatoes.

In a non-stick pan heat 1 teaspoon of vegetable oil and Sauté shredded potatoes till cooked slightly for 4 minutes.

Cool it down and transfer the potatoes to a plate. Add corn flour, salt, pepper, garlic and onion powder and chili flakes and mix together roughly.

Spread over the plate and pat it firmly with your fingers. Refrigerate it for about 20 minutes.

Preheat air fryer at 1800C, take out the now refrigerated potato and divide into equal pieces with a knife.

Brush the wire basket of the air fryer with little oil. Place the hash brown pieces in the basket and fry for about 15 minutes at 1800C.

Take out the basket and flip the hash browns at 6 minutes so that they are air fried uniformly. Serve it hot with ketchup

Chapter 9. Gourmet Lunches

Lunch Egg Rolls

Preparation time: 25 Minutes

Servings: 4

Ingredients

½ cup mushrooms

½ cup carrots

½ cup zucchini

2 green onions

2 tbsp. soy sauce

8 egg roll

1egg

1 tbsp. Cornstarch

Instructions

Mix carrots with soy sauce, zucchini, green onions and mushrooms in a bowl. Stir.

Organize egg roll wrappers on a surface. Divide veggie mix on each. Roll well.

Mix cornstarch plus egg in a bowl. Whisk well. Brush eggs rolls with this mix.

Seal edges. Place all rolls in preheated air fryer. Cook for 15 minutes at 370°F.

Arrange them on a platter. Serve.

Veggie Toast

Preparation time: 25 Minutes

Servings: 4

Ingredients:

1 red bell pepper

1 cup cremimi mushrooms

2 greenonions

1 tbsp. olive oil

4 breadslices

2 tbsp. butter

½ cup goat cheese

Directions:

Mix mushrooms and red bell pepper in a bowl squash. Add oil and green onions. Toss. Transfer to air fryer. Cook them for 10 minutes at 350°F. Transfer to a bowl.

On bread slices, spread butter. Place them in airfryer. Cook for 5 minutes them at 350°F.

Divide veggie mix on the bread slices. Top using crumbled cheese. Serve.

Stuffed Mushrooms

Preparation time: 30 minutes

Servings: 4

Ingredients

4 big Portobello mushroom caps

1 tbsp. olive oil

¼ cup ricotta cheese

5 tbsp. parmesan

1 cup spinach

1/3 cup bread crumbs

¼ tsp. rosemary

Directions:

Rub mushrooms caps with the oil. Place them in your air fryer's basket. Cook for 2 minutes at 350°F.

Mix half of the parmesan with bread crumbs, rosemary, spinach and ricotta in a bowl. Stir.

Stuff mushrooms with this mix. Drizzle with parmesan. Place in your air fryer's basket. Cook for 10 minutes at 350°F.

Divide on plates and serve.

Quick Lunch Pizzas

Preparation time: 17 Minutes

Servings: 4

Ingredients

4 pitas

1 tablespoon olive oil

¾ cup pizza sauce

4 ounces jarred mushrooms

½ tsp. basil

2 green onions

2 cup mozzarella

1 cup grape tomatoes

Directions:

On each pita bread, spread pizza sauce. Drizzle basil and green onions. Divide mushrooms top with cheese.

Assemble pita pizzas in air fryer. Cook for 7 minutes at 400°F.

Top pizza with tomato slices. Divide among plates. Serve.

Lunch Gnocchi

Preparation time: 10 Minutes

Servings: 4

Ingredients

1 yellow onion

1 tablespoon olive oil

3 garliccloves

16 oz. gnocchi

¼ cup parmesan

8 oz. spinach pesto

Instructions

Grease air fryer's pan with olive oil. Include garlic, onion and gnocchi. Toss. Place pan in air fryer. Cook for 10 minutes at 400°F.

Add pesto. Toss. Cook for 7 minutes at 350°F.

Divide among plates. Serve.

Lunch Gnocchi

Preparation time: 10 Minutes

Servings: 4

Ingredients:

1 yellow onion

1 tbsp.olive oil

3 garlic cloves

16 ounces' gnocchi

¼ cup parmesan

8 oz. Spinach pesto

Directions:

Lubricate air fryer's pan with olive oil. Include garlic, onion and gnocchi. Toss. Place pan in air fryer. Cook for 10 minutes at 400°F.

Include pesto. Toss. Cook for 7 minutes at 350°F.

Divide among plates. Serve.

Tuna and Zucchini Tortillas

Preparation time: 10 Minutes

Servings: 4

Ingredients:

4 corn tortillas

4 tbsp. butter

6 oz. canned tuna

1 cup zucchini

1/3 cupmayonnaise

2 tbsp. mustard

1 cup cheddar cheese

Directions:

Spreadbutter on tortillas. Put in air fryer's basket. Cook for 3 minutes at 400°F.

Mix mustard with mayo, zucchini and tuna in a bowl. Stir.

Mix on each tortilla. Garnish with cheese. Position in your air fryer's basket. Cook for 4 minutes at 400°F.

Serve.

Squash Fritters

Preparation time: 10Minutes

Servings: 4

Ingredients:

3 oz. cream cheese

1 egg

½ tsp. oregano

Black pepper and a pinch of salt

1 yellow summer squash

1/3 cupcarrot

2/3 cupbread crumbs

2 tbsp. olive oil

Directions:

Mix cream cheese with pepper, salt, egg, oregano, carrot, bread crumbs and squash in a bowl. Stir.

Make medium patties from this mix. Brush them with oil

Arrange squash patties in air fryer. Cook for 7 minutes at 400° F

Serve.

Lunch Shrimp Croquettes

Preparation time: 18minutes

Servings: 4

Ingredients:

2/3-pound shrimp

1 ½ cups bread crumbs

1 egg

2 tbsp. lemon juice

3 green onions

½ tsp. basil

Salt and black pepper to

2 tbsp. olive oil

Directions:

Mix egg and half of the bread crumbs with lemon juice in a bowl. Stir.

Add basil, green onions, pepper, shrimp and salt. Stir.

Mix the rest of the bread crumbs with the oil in a separate bowl. Toss well.

Make round balls from shrimp mix. Dredge in bread crumbs. Put them in heated air fryer and cook for 8 minutes at 400°F.

Serve.

Lunch Special Pancake

Preparation time: 10 Minutes

Servings: 2

Ingredients

1 tbsp. butter

3 eggs

½ cup flour

½ cup milk

1 cup salsa

1 cup small shrimp

Instructions

Heat air fryer at 400°F. Include 1 tbsp. butter. Melt it.

Mix eggs with milk and in a bowl. Whisk. Pour into air fryer's pan. Cook for 12 minutes at 350°F. Transfer to a plate.

Mix salsa with shrimp in a bowl. Stir.

Serve.

Scallops and Dill

Preparation time: 15 Minutes

Servings: 4

Ingredients

1 lb. sea scallops

1 tbsp. lemon juice

1 tsp. dill

2 tsp. olive oil

Black pepper and salt

Instructions

Mix scallops with oil, dill, pepper, lemon juice and salt in air fryer. Close. Cook for 5 minutes at 360° F.

Dispose uncovered ones. Divide dill sauce and scallops on plates. Serve.

Chicken Sandwiches

Preparation time: 20 minutes

Servings: 4

Ingredients:

2 chicken breasts, boneless, skinless

1 red onion

1 red bell pepper

½ cup Italian seasoning

½ tsp. thyme

2 cups butter lettuce

4 pita pockets

1 cup cherry tomatoes

1 tablespoon olive oil

Instructions

Mix chicken with bell pepper, onion, oil and Italian seasoning. Toss. Cook for 10 minutes at 380°F.

Place chicken mix into a bowl. Include butter lettuce, cherry tomatoes and thyme. Toss. Stuff pita pockets with this mix. Serve.

Hot Bacon Sandwiches

Preparation time: 10 Minutes

Servings: 4

Ingredients

1/3 cup bbq sauce

2 tbsp.honey

8 bacon slices

1 red bell pepper

1 yellow bell pepper

3 pita pockets

1¼ cup butter lettuce leaves

2 tomatoes

Instructions

Mix bbq with honey with sauce in a bowl. Whisk.

Brush all bell peppers and bacon with this mix. Put them in air fryer. Cook at 350°F for 4 minutes.

Stuff pita pockets with lettuce, bacon mix and tomatoes, spread the rest of the bbq sauce and serve for lunch.

Chapter 10.   Traditional Dinners For Beginners

Air-fryer Tofu Satay

Ingredients:

1 block tofu, extra firm

2 tbsp. soy sauce

2 tsp ginger garlic paste

1 tsp sriracha sauce

1 tbsp. maple syrup + lime juice

Directions:

Mix the maple syrup with lime juice, ginger garlic paste, sriracha, and soy sauce in a food processor or blender. Blend it until smooth.

Cut the tofu into strips. Add the puree over the strips and let it marinate for 15 to 30 minutes.

Soak 6 bamboo skewers in water while the tofu marinates.

With a wire cutter, cut each skewer into two, as a full skewer will not fit inside the air-fryer.

Skewer one strip of tofu to each bamboo stick. Peirce it through the uncut side of the skewer.

Place the skewers in the air-fryer. Set the temperature to 370 F and let it cook for 15 minutes. You do not have to toss the contents.

Serve with peanut butter sauce.

Sticky-Sweet BBQ Tofu

Ingredients:

1 ½ cups BBQ sauce

1 block tofu, extra firm

Oil for greasing

Directions:

Set the temperature to 400 F and preheat the air-fryer.

Press down the tofu and slice it into 1" cubes.

Place them on a greased baking sheet.

Apply a coat of BBQ sauce and let it cook in the air-fryer for 20 minutes. Keep it aside.

Add ½ cup of BBQ sauce into a glass saucepan. The sauce should evenly spread in the pan. Place the cooked tofu cubes on top and add another layer of the sauce on it.

Transfer them to the air-fryer again and let it cook for 30 minutes.

Enjoy!

Veggie Bowl

Ingredients

4 cups Brussel sprouts

6 cups sweet potato

2 tsp garlic powder

2 tbsp. soy sauce, low sodium

Cooking spray

Directions:

Place the sweet potatoes in the air-fryer. Add a light layer of oil for tossing.

Top it with 1 tsp of garlic powder and toss.

Set the temperature to 400 F and cook for 15 minutes. Toss after 5 minutes.

Transfer the Brussels sprouts to the cooking basket and spray a layer of oil and the remaining garlic powder. Toss them well and cook at 400 F for 5 minutes.

Drizzle some soy sauce and shake to coat the vegetables evenly.

Set to the same temperature and cook for 5 minutes. Check it when it hits 2 minutes and toss the contents.

Cooking time will depend on the vegetable. Once the vegetables are done they will be soft and brown.

Air fried Fish skin

Ingredients:

½ pound salmon skin

2 tbsp. heart-healthy oil

Salt and pepper, as needed

Directions:

Set the temperature to 400 F and preheat the air-fryer for 5 minutes.

Make sure the salmon skin is patted dry.

In a large mixing bowl, add everything and combine well.

Transfer the ingredients to the air-fryer basket and close it

Allow it to cook for 10 minutes at a temperature of 400 F.

Shake the items halfway through the cooking time, to make sure that the skin is cooked evenly.

Baked Thai fish

Ingredients:

1 pound cod fillet

1 tbsp. lime juice

¼ cup of coconut milk

Salt and pepper, as needed

Directions:

Cut the cod fillet into small pieces.

Set the temperature to 325 F and preheat the fryer for 5 minutes.

Add all the ingredients to a baking dish and transfer it to an air-fryer.

Let it cook for 20 minutes at a temperature of 325 F.

Enjoy!

Oven Braised Corned Beef

Ingredients:

1 medium onion, chopped

4 cups of water

2 tbsp. Dijon mustard

3 pounds corned beef brisket

Directions:

Set the temperature to 400 F and preheat the air-fryer for 5 minutes.

Slice the brisket to chunks

Add all the ingredients to a baking tray that fits inside the air-fryer.

Let it cook for 50 minutes at a temperature of 400 F.

Enjoy!

Crispy Keto Pork Bites

Ingredients:

1 medium onion

½ pound pork belly

4 tbsp. coconut cream

1 tbsp. butter

Salt & pepper, to taste

Directions:

Slice the pork belly into even and thin strips

The onion has to be diced.

Transfer all the ingredients into a mixing bowl and allow it to marinate in the fridge for the next two hours.

Set the temperature to 350 F and preheat the air-fryer for 5 minutes.

Keep the pork strips inside the air-fryer and let it cook for 25 minutes at a temperature of 350 F.

Enjoy!

Soy and Garlic Mushrooms

Ingredients:

2 pounds mushrooms

2 garlic cloves

¼ cup coconut aminos

3 tbsp. olive oil

Directions:

Transfer all the ingredients to a dish and combine until well incorporated.

Let it marinate for 2 hours in a fridge

Set the temperature to 350 F and preheat for 5 minutes.

Transfer the mushrooms to a heatproof dish that can fit in an air-fryer

Let it cook for 20 minutes at a temperature of 350 F.

Enjoy!

Crack Chicken

Ingredients:

1 block cream cheese

4 chicken breast

8 slices of bacon

¼ cup olive oil

Salt and pepper

Direction:

Set the temperature to 350 F and let the air-fryer preheat for 5 minutes

In a baking dish that can fit the air-fryer, place the chicken.

Apply the cream cheese and olive oil on it. Fry the bacon and crumble it on top of the chicken.

Season as needed.

Transfer the dish into the air-fryer and cook it for 25 minutes at a temperature of 350 F.

Enjoy!

Portobello Mushrooms and Steak Tips in an Air Fryer

Preparation Time: 5 minutes

Cooking Time: 10 minutes

Servings: 2

Ingredients:

Olive oil: ¼ cup

Coconut aminos: 1 tablespoon

Montreal steak seasoning: 2 teaspoons

Garlic powder: ½ teaspoon

Steaks: 2 strips (make ¾-inch pieces

Portobello mushrooms: 4 ounces (quartered

Directions:

Start by preparing the marinade for the steaks. To do this, take a small bowl and add the coconut aminos, olive oil, garlic powder, and steak seasoning. Mix well to combine.

Add the steak pieces to the mixture and let them sit in the marinade for about 15 minutes.

In the meantime, preheat the air fryer by setting the temperature to 390°F.

Take the basket out of the air fryer and line the grill bottom with parchment paper.

Remove the steak strips from the marinade and place them in the basket of the air fryer. Also, add the portobello mushrooms

Let the steak and mushrooms cook for about 5 minutes. Take the basket out and toss the mushrooms and steak around. Cook for another 4 minutes.

Transfer the contents of the basket onto a plate and serve hot.

Nutrition: Proteins: 41 g Carbohydrates: 4.9 g Fat: 40.1 g

Air-Fried Classic Pork Chops

Preparation Time: 10 minutes

Cooking Time: 20 minutes

Servings: 4

Ingredients:

Parmesan cheese: ½ cup (grated

Paprika: 1 teaspoon

Garlic powder: 1 teaspoon

Kosher salt: 1 teaspoon

Dried parsley: 1 teaspoon

Ground black pepper: ½ teaspoon

Pork chops (center-cut: 4 (5 ounces

Extra virgin olive oil: 2 tablespoons

Arugula leaves for garnishing

Lemon (cut in wedges for garnishing

Directions:

Start by preheating the air fryer to 380°F.

Take a shallow dish and add the parmesan cheese, garlic powder, paprika, salt, pepper, and parsley. Mix well to combine.

Drizzle the olive oil over the pork chops and ensure that they are well coated.

Dredge the pork chops in the parmesan mixture. Make sure that both sides are evenly coated.

Take the air fryer basket and place 2 pork chops inside it. Let them cook for about 5 minutes. Remove the basket and flip them over. Cook for another 5 minutes. Repeat the process with the remaining chops.

Transfer the cooked pork chops onto a wooden chopping board. Let them rest for 5 minutes.

Place them on a plate and serve them with arugula leaves and lemon wedges.

Nutrition: Proteins: 35.3 g Carbohydrates: 1.5 g Fat: 16.6 g

Air-Fried Sexy Meatloaf

Preparation Time: 10 minutes

Cooking Time: 45 minutes

Servings: 4

Ingredients:

Ground pork: ½ pound

Ground veal: ½ pound

Egg: 1 (large

Fresh cilantro: ¼ cup (chopped

Bread crumbs: ¼ cup (gluten-free

Spring onions: 2 medium (diced

Freshly ground black pepper: ½ teaspoon

Sriracha salt: ½ teaspoon

Ketchup: ½ cup

Chipotle chili sauce: 2 teaspoons (gluten-free

Olive oil: 1 teaspoon

Blackstrap molasses: 1 teaspoon

Directions:

Start by preheating the air fryer by setting the temperature to 400°F.

Take a baking dish (nonstick that can easily fit inside the basket of the air fryer. Add the veal and pork and mix well to combine.

In the center of the veal and pork mixture, make a well. Add the egg, bread crumbs, cilantro, black pepper, spring onions, and Sriracha salt. Use your hands to mix all the ingredients together.

Mold the mixture in the shape of a loaf in the nonstick baking dish.

Place the baking dish inside the air fryer basket and let the meatloaf cook for about 25 minutes.

In the meantime, take a small bowl and add the chipotle chili sauce, ketchup, molasses, and olive oil. Mix well using a whisk. Set aside

Remove the basket and top the meatloaf with the ketchup and chipotle mixture. Make sure you completely cover the top of the meatloaf.

Place the basket in the air fryer again and cook for about 7 more minutes.

Turn off the air fryer and let the meatloaf rest inside it for about 5 minutes.

Remove the basket and transfer the meatloaf onto a wooden board. Let it rest for about 5 minutes.

Cut the meatloaf into slices and serve hot.

Notes:

- You can replace the Sriracha with chipotle sauce.

- You can also opt for crumbs from regular bread instead of crumbs from gluten-free bread.

Nutrition: Proteins: 22.1 g Carbohydrates: 13.3 g Fat: 14.4 g

Air- Fried Jerk Pork Skewers Served with Mango and Black Bean Salsa

Preparation Time: 30 minutes

Cooking Time: 10 minutes

Servings: 4

Ingredients:

Jamaican Jerk Seasoning:

White sugar: 2 tablespoons

Onion powder: 4 ½ teaspoons

Dried thyme: 4 ½ teaspoons (crushed

Ground allspice: 1 tablespoon

Freshly ground black pepper: 1 tablespoon

Cayenne pepper: 1 ½ teaspoons

Salt: 1 ½ teaspoons

Ground nutmeg: ¾ teaspoon

Ground cloves: ¼ teaspoon

Shredded coconut: ¼ cup

Pork tenderloin: 1 (1 pound

Bamboo skewers: 4

Vegetable oil: 1 tablespoon

Mango: 1 peeled, seeded, and chopped

Black beans (rinsed and drained: ½ can (15 ounces

Red onion (finely chopped: ¼ cup

Fresh lime juice: 2 tablespoons

Honey: 1 tablespoon

Fresh cilantro (chopped: 1 tablespoon

Salt: ¼ teaspoon

Black pepper (freshly ground: ⅛ teaspoon

Directions:

Start by soaking the skewers in water for about 30 minutes.

In the meantime, prepare the seasoning for the pork. Take a small bowl and add the sugar, thyme, onion powder, allspice, cayenne pepper, salt, black pepper, cloves, and nutmeg.

Save 1 tablespoon of seasoning for the recipe and store the rest for future use.

Take the pork tenderloin and cut it in 1 ½-inch cubes. Add these cubes and coconut to the reserved spice mixture. Combine by mixing well.

Preheat the air fryer by setting the temperature to 350°F.

Remove the skewers from the water and start threading the pork chunks on the prepared skewers.

Grease the pork generously with oil using a brush. Sprinkle the pork with the spice mixture. Make sure all sides are coated evenly.

Place the threaded pork skewers in the basket of the air fryer. Cook for about 5-7 minutes.

While the pork is cooking, take the mango and peel off the skin. Remove the seed and dice the flesh into small cubes.

In a medium-sized bowl, add 1/3 of the diced mango and mash it to make a smooth paste. Add the remaining diced mango, red onion, black beans, honey, lime juice, salt, pepper, and cilantro. Mix well to combine.

Once cooked, remove the skewered pork from the air fryer basket and place it on a platter. Serve with salsa.

Nutrition: Proteins: 22.3 g Carbohydrates: 34.6 g Fat: 10.8 g

Pork Meatballs in an Air Fryer

Preparation Time: 10 minutes

Cooking Time: 20 minutes

Ingredients:

Ground pork: 12 ounces

Ground Italian sausage: 8 ounces

Panko bread crumbs: ½ cup

Egg: 1

Salt: 1 teaspoon

Dried parsley: 1 teaspoon

Paprika: ½ teaspoon

Directions:

Start by preheating the air fryer by setting the temperature to 350°F.

Take a large bowl and add the pork, bread crumbs, sausage, salt, egg, paprika, and parsley. Mix well and make sure it is properly combined.

Make 12 equal-sized meatballs. This can be done by using a scoop. Mold them into round balls

Take a baking sheet and place all the meatballs on it. Grease the air fryer basket lightly and place all the meatballs into the basket. Let them cook for about 8 minutes. Remove the basket and shake it well. Cook for another 2 minutes.

Transfer the meatballs onto a plate and leave them to rest for 5 minutes.

Nutrition: Proteins: 8.5 g Carbohydrates: 3.8 g Fat: 8.1 g

Breaded Pork Chops in an Air Fryer

Preparation Time: 10 minutes

Cooking Time: 10 minutes

Servings: 4

Ingredients:

Pork chops (center-cut and boneless: 4

Cajun seasoning: 1 teaspoon

Garlic-and-cheese-flavored croutons: 1 ½ cups

Eggs: 2

Cooking spray

Directions:

Start by preheating the air fryer by setting the temperature to 390°F.

Take a plate and transfer the Cajun seasoning to it. Take 1 pork chop and coat it with the seasoning. Make sure both sides are evenly coated. Repeat the process with the remaining chops.

In a food processor, pulse the flavored croutons until the consistency is fine. Once done, empty them onto a shallow dish.

Take another shallow dish and dip each pork chops into the eggs. Then coat them in the crouton crumble evenly on all sides. Set them aside on a plate.

Take the air fryer basket and grease it using the cooking spray. Place 2 chops inside the basket and cook them for about 5 minutes. Flip over the chops and lightly mist them using a cooking spray. Cook for another 5 minutes. Repeat the process with the remaining pork chops.

Once done, transfer the cooked chops onto a serving platter and serve hot.

Nutrition: Proteins: 44.7 g Carbohydrates −10 g Fat: 18.1 g

Pork Ribs in an Air Fryer with Ginger Glaze

Preparation Time: 20 minutes

Cooking Time: 30 minutes

Servings: 6

Ingredients:

Pork ribs (country-style: 2 pounds

Vegetable oil: 2 tablespoons

Salt: ¼ teaspoon

Black pepper (freshly ground: ¼ teaspoon

Vegetable oil: 2 teaspoons

Shallot (finely chopped: 1

Chili sauce: 1/3 cup

Apricot preserves: 1/3 cup

Soy sauce (reduced-sodium: 1 tablespoon

Fresh ginger (grated: 1 teaspoon

Ground chipotle pepper: ⅛ teaspoon

Fresh chives (chopped: For garnishing

Directions:

Start by preheating the air fryer by setting the temperature to 350°F.

Also, preheat an oven by setting the temperature to 200°F.

Gently brush the ribs with 2 tablespoons of vegetable oil. Season the ribs with pepper and salt.

Take an air fryer basket and arrange half of the ribs in it. Place the basket in the air fryer and cook for about 15 to 20 minutes. To determine whether the ribs are properly cooked, insert an instant-read thermometer into the thickest part of the ribs. The temperature should be 145°F.

Once done, take a baking dish and transfer the cooked ribs to the oven. Change the setting of the oven to keep it warm. In the meantime, cook the remaining pork ribs by following the above procedure.

While the second batch of pork ribs is being cooked, prepare the ginger glaze. For this, place a small saucepan over medium flame. Pour 2 teaspoons of vegetable oil and let it heat. Add the finely chopped shallots and keep stirring until they turn pink. This will take about 3 minutes. Add the apricot preserve, chili sauce, ginger, soy sauce, and chipotle pepper. Keep stirring. Cook for 3-5 minutes.

Remove the pork ribs from the air fryer basket and the oven and transfer them to a platter. Generously brush them with the prepared ginger glaze. Sprinkle chives over the ribs and serve hot.

Nutrition: Proteins: 16.3 g Carbohydrates: 17 g Fat: 22.9 g

Air Fryer Pork Burger Patties

Preparation Time: 10 minutes

Cooking Time: 10 minutes

Servings: 4

Ingredients:

Ground beef (16 ounces: 1 package

Red onion: ½ (diced

Minced garlic: 1 teaspoon

Salt: 1 teaspoon

Black pepper (freshly ground: 1 teaspoon

Worcestershire sauce: 1 teaspoon

Hot English mustard: 1 teaspoon

Directions:

Start by preheating the air fryer by setting the temperature to 350°F.

In a large mixing bowl, add the beef, minced garlic, red onion, English mustard sauce, Worcestershire sauce, pepper, and salt. Mix well to combine.

Divide the beef mixture into 4 equal portions. Mold each portion into a round ball and then make a flat patty using your hands. Repeat with the remaining portions of the beef mixture.

Place the prepared patties in the air fryer basket. Cook them in the air fryer for 10 minutes.

Nutrition: Proteins: 19.4 g Carbohydrates: 2.2 g Fat: 13.8 g

Chapter 11.   Gourmet Dinners

Light & Crispy Okra

Cooking Time: 10 minutes

Servings: 4

Ingredients:

3 cups okra, wash and dry

1 teaspoon fresh lemon juice

1 teaspoon coriander

3 tablespoons gram flour

2 teaspoons red chili powder

1 teaspoon dry mango powder

1 teaspoon cumin powder

Sea salt to taste

Directions:

Cut the top of okra then cut a deep horizontal cut in each okra and set aside. In a bowl, combine gram flour, salt, lemon juice, and all the spices. Add a little water in gram flour mixture and make a thick batter. Fill batter in each okra and place in the air fryer basket. Spray okra with cooking spray. Preheat your air fryer to 350°Fahrenheit for 5-minutes. Air fry the stuffed okra for 10-minutes or until lightly golden brown. Serve and enjoy!

Nutrition: Calories: 56, Total Fat: 0.8g, Carbs: 9g, Protein: 2g

Chili Rellenos

Cooking Time: 35 minutes

Servings: 5

Ingredients:

2 cans of green chili peppers

1 cup of Monterey Jack cheese

½ cup milk

1 can tomato sauce

2 tablespoons almond flour

1 can evaporated milk

1 cup of cheddar cheese, shredded

2 large beaten eggs

Directions:

Preheat the air fryer to 350°Fahrenheit. Spray a baking dish with cooking spray. Take half of the chilies and arrange them in the baking dish. Sprinkle the chilies with half of the cheese and cover with the rest of chilies. In a medium bowl, combine milk, eggs, flour and pour the mixture over the chilies. Air fry for 25-minutes. Remove the chilies from the Air fryer pour tomato sauce over them and cook them for an additional 10-minutes. Remove them from air fryer and top with remaining cheese.

Nutrition: Calories: 282, Total Fat: 6.2g, Carbs: 7.4g, Protein: 5g

Persian Mushrooms

Cooking Time: 20 minutes

Servings: 3

Ingredients:

6 Portobello large mushrooms

3-ounces of softened butter

1 cup parmesan cheese, grated

A pinch of black pepper

A pinch of sea salt

1 tablespoon parsley, fresh, chopped

2 cloves of garlic

2 large shallots

Directions:

Preheat your air fryer to 390°Fahrenheit. Clean the mushrooms and remove the stems. Slice the shallots and garlic cloves. Now, place the mushroom stems, garlic, shallots, parsley and softened butter into a blender. Arrange the caps of the mushrooms in the air fryer basket. Stuff the caps with the mixture and sprinkle tops with parmesan cheese. Cook for 20-minutes. Serve warm and enjoy!

Nutrition: Calories: 278, Total Fat: 9.8g, Carbs: 7.2g, Protein: 4.3g

Air Fried Chicken Cordon Bleu

Cooking Time: 45 minutes

Servings: 4

Ingredients:

4 skinless and boneless chicken breasts

4 slices of ham

4 slices of Swiss cheese

3 tablespoons almond flour

1 cup of heavy whipping cream

1 teaspoon of chicken bouillon granules

½ cup dry white wine

5 tablespoons butter

1 teaspoon paprika

Directions:

Preheat your air fryer to 390°Fahrenheit. Pound the chicken breasts and put a slice of ham and Swiss cheese on each breast. Fold over edges of the chicken; cover the filling and secure the edges with toothpicks. In a bowl, combine flour, and paprika. Coat chicken with this mixture. Set the air fryer to cook the chicken for 15-minutes. In a large skillet, heat the butter, bouillon, and wine then reduce heat to low. Remove the chicken from air fryer and add it to the skillet. Allow the components to simmer for around 30-minutes. Serve warm and enjoy!

Nutrition: Calories: 389, Total Fat: 12.7g, Carbs: 9.2g, Protein: 32.4g

Chicken Noodles

Cooking Time: 25 minutes

Servings: 4

Ingredients:

4 chicken breasts

1 teaspoon rosemary

1 teaspoon allspices

1 teaspoon red pepper

1 teaspoon tomato paste

1 tablespoon butter

5 cups chicken broth

Sesame seeds for garnish

For Noodles:

2 beaten eggs

½ teaspoon salt

2 cups almond flour

Directions:

Preheat your air fryer to 350°Fahrenheit. Coat the chicken with 1 tablespoon of butter, salt, and pepper. Arrange the chicken breasts in the air fryer basket and cook for 20-minutes. For the noodles, combine egg, salt, and flour to make a dough. Put the dough on a floured surface knead it for a few minutes then cover it and set it aside for 30-minutes. Roll the dough on a floured surface. When the dough is thin, cut it into thin strips and allow them to dry for an hour. Meanwhile, take the chicken out of the air fryer and place aside. Boil the chicken broth and add the noodles, tomato paste and red pepper, cook for 5-minutes. Add the spices and stir noodles. Add salt and pepper to taste. Serve noodles with air fried chicken and garnish with sesame seeds. Serve hot and enjoy!

Nutrition: Calories: 387, Total Fat: 12.7g, Carbs: 6.8g, Protein: 38.2g

Mushroom & Herb Stuffed Pork Chops

Cooking Time: 52 minutes

Servings: 5

Ingredients:

5 thick pork chops

7 mushrooms, chopped

1 pinch of herbs

1 tablespoon almond flour

1 tablespoon lemon juice

Salt and black pepper to taste

Directions:

Preheat your air fryer to 325°Fahrenheit. Season both sides of meat with salt and pepper. Arrange the chops in the air fryer and cook for 15-minutes at 350°Fahrenheit. Cook the mushrooms for 3-minutes in a pan over medium heat and stir in lemon juice. Add the flour and herbs to pan and stir. Cook the mixture for 4-minutes, then set aside. Cut five pieces of foil for each chop. O every piece of foil put a chop in the middle and cover it with mushroom mixture. Now, carefully fold the foil and seal around the chop. Place chops back into air fryer and cook for an additional 30-minutes. Serve with salad.

Nutrition: Calories: 389, Total Fat: 14.2g, Carbs: 9.2g, Protein: 38.5g

Roasted Lamb with Pumpkin

Cooking Time: 33 minutes

Servings: 2

Ingredients:

1 lamb rack

1 tablespoon Dijon mustard

2-ounces of almond breadcrumbs

2 tablespoons herbs, chopped

Salt and pepper to taste

1 tablespoon olive oil

1-ounce parmesan cheese, grated

1-medium pumpkin

1-lemon zest

Directions:

Preheat your air fryer to 390°Fahrenheit for 3-minutes. Pat the lamb dry using a towel. Remove the fat and rub the meat with mustard. Blitz the breadcrumbs with herbs, parmesan cheese, lemon zest, and seasonings. Season the joint. Place the meat into air fryer and roast for 15-minutes. For the pumpkin wedges, start by peeling and coring the pumpkin; then coat it with oil. Season the pumpkin then coat it with oil and place it aside. Take the lamb meat out of the air fryer and place it in serving the dish. Add pumpkin wedges to air fryer and roast them for 15-minutes. Once the pumpkin wedges are done, serve with meat!

Nutrition: Calories: 386, Total Fat: 13.2g, Carbs: 9.3g, Protein: 37.3g

Liver Curry

Cooking Time: 35 minutes

Servings: 3

Ingredients:

Coriander leaves

4 drops of liquid stevia

½ teaspoon ground coriander

½ teaspoon turmeric

1 teaspoon ginger

1 clove of garlic, minced

1 large tomato, chopped

1 onion, sliced

½ lb. of beef liver

½ teaspoon of Garam Masala

1 teaspoon cumin powder

Directions:

In a pan, fry the onion over medium heat for 5-minutes. Add the garlic and grated ginger and stir. Add the powdered spices, and fry for additional 3-minutes. Meanwhile, season the liver with salt and pepper. Place the liver in the air fryer and cook it for 15-minutes at 350°Fahrenheit. Remove the liver from the air fryer and transfer it to the skillet. Add the chopped tomato, and stevia and a little bit of water, and cook for a few more minutes. Serve and garnish with coriander.

Nutrition: Calories: 292, Total Fat: 11.2g, Carbs: 8.2g, Protein: 42g

Minced Beef Kebab Skewers

Cooking Time: 25 minutes

Servings: 2

Ingredients:

½ lb. of minced beef

½ large onion, chopped

1 medium green chili

½ teaspoon chili powder

1 clove of garlic, minced

1 pinch of ginger

1 teaspoon Garam Masala

3 tablespoons of pork rinds

Directions:

Grate the ginger and garlic. Chop and deseed the chili. Chop the onion. Mix the ginger, chili, and onion with the minced beef. Add the powdered spices. Add a few pork rinds and salt. Shape the beef into fat sausages around short wooden skewers. Set the skewers aside for an hour, then cook them in your preheated air fryer for 25-minutes at 350°Fahrenheit.

Pomfret Fish Fry

Cooking Time: 15-minutes

Servings: 5

Ingredients:

4 onions

3 lbs. of silver Pomfret

Salt and black pepper to taste

2 tablespoons olive oil

2 teaspoons lemon juice

3 pinches of cumin powder

¾ teaspoons of ginger

3 pinches of red chili powder

1 tablespoon turmeric powder

1 teaspoon garlic paste

Directions:

Wash the fish with clean water and soak it in lemon juice to remove any unpleasant smell. After 30-minutes, take the fish out and wash it with clean water. Draw diagonal shaped slits on the fish. Combine the black pepper, salt, lemon juice, garlic paste, and turmeric powder. Rub the mixture inside and outside of fish and leave it in the fridge for 30-minutes to absorb the seasoning. Add the fish to air fryer basket with 2 tablespoons olive oil and cook for 12-minutes at 340°Fahrenheit.

Nutrition: Calories: 278, Total Fat: 8.6g, Carbs: 7.4g, Protein: 32g

Cedar Planked Salmon

Cooking Time: 15 minutes

Servings: 6

Ingredients:

4 untreated cedar planks

½ cup olive oil

1 ½ tablespoons of rice vinegar

1 teaspoon sesame oil

2 lbs. of salmon fillets, skin removed

1 teaspoon garlic, minced

1 tablespoon ginger root, fresh, grated

¼ cup green onions, chopped

½ cup soy sauce

Directions:

Start by soaking the cedar planks for 2-hours. Take a shallow baking dish and stir in the olive oil, the rice vinegar, the sesame oil, soy sauce, ginger, and green onions. Place the salmon fillets in the prepared marinade for at least 20-minutes. Place the planks in the basket of your air fryer. Cook the salmon fillets for 15-minutes at 360°Fahrenheit.

Nutrition: Calories: 273, Total Fat: 7.5g, Carbs: 5.2g, Protein: 34.2g

Crested Halibut

Cooking Time: 30 minutes

Servings: 4

Ingredients:

4 halibut fillets

¾ cup of pork rinds

½ cup of parsley, fresh, chopped

¼ cup dill, fresh, chopped

¼ cup chives, fresh, chopped

1 tablespoon olive oil

1 teaspoon lemon zest, finely grated

Sea salt and black pepper to taste

Directions:

Preheat your air fryer to 390°Fahrenheit. In a mixing bowl, combine the pork rinds, parsley, dill, chives, olive oil, lemon zest, sea salt and black pepper. Rinse the halibut fillets and dry them on a paper towel. Arrange the halibut fillets and dry them on a paper towel. Arrange the halibut fillets onto a baking sheet. Spoon the pork rind crumb mixture onto fish fillets. Lightly press the mixture on the fillets. Bake the fillets in your preheated air fryer basket for 30-minutes. Serve warm.

Nutrition: Calories: 272, Total Fat: 10.3g, Carbs: 9.4g, Protein: 32.2g

Creamy Halibut

Cooking Time: 20 minutes

Servings: 6

Ingredients:

2 lbs. of halibut fillets, cut into 6 pieces

1 teaspoon dill weed, dried

½ cup light sour cream

½ cup light mayonnaise

4-chopped green onions

Directions:

Preheat the air fryer to 390°Fahrenheit. Season the halibut with salt and pepper. In a bowl, mix the onions, sour cream, mayonnaise, and dill. Spread the onion mixture evenly over the halibut fillets. Cook in air fryer for 20-minutes. Serve warm.

Nutrition: Calories: 286, Total Fat: 11.3g, Carbs: 6.9, Protein: 29.8g

Air Fried Catfish

Cooking Time: 20 minutes

Servings: 2

Ingredients:

5 catfish filets

1 pinch of salt

1 teaspoon garlic powder

1 teaspoon crab seasoning

1 cup almond flour

2 tablespoons olive oil for spraying

2 tablespoons hot sauce

1 cup buttermilk

Black pepper as needed

Directions:

Season catfish fillets on both sides with salt and pepper. In a dish, combine the buttermilk with hot sauce. Add the catfish fillets and cover them with liquid. Let the ingredients soak while you prepare the rest of the ingredients. Whisk the flour, crab seasoning, and garlic powder in a casserole dish. Remove the catfish from the buttermilk and allow excess liquid to drip off. Dredge the catfish on both sides in the flour mixture. Place fillets into air fryer and drizzle with oil. Cook at 390°Fahrenheit for 15-minutes. When cooking is completed remove basket and gently turn the fillets over, spray some oil on them, and cook for an additional 5-minutes.

Nutrition: Calories: 283, Total Fat: 8.6g, Carbs: 6.5g, Protein: 34.3g

Air Fried Spinach Fish

Cooking Time: 12 minutes

Servings: 2

Ingredients:

4-ounces of spinach leaves

1 large egg, beaten

2 tablespoons olive oil

2 cups almond flour

2 white fish fillets

Pinch of sea salt

Black pepper to taste

Directions:

In a deep bowl, place the beaten egg, almond flour, sea salt, black pepper, and spinach leaves. Marinate the fish for 2-hours in the fridge. Transfer the fish to air fryer and cook for 12-minutes at 370°Fahrenheit. Serve with lemon slices.

Nutrition: Calories: 286, Total Fat: 11.2g, Carbs: 5.2g, Protein: 29.7g

Roly Poly Air Fried White Fish

Cooking Time: 10 minutes

Servings: 4

Ingredients:

4 lbs. of white fish fillets

2 ½ teaspoons of sea salt

4 mushrooms, sliced

1 teaspoon liquid stevia

2 tablespoons of Chinese winter pickle

2 tablespoons of vinegar

2 teaspoons chili powder

2 onions, thinly sliced

1 cup vegetable stock

2 tablespoons soy sauce

Directions:

Fill the fish fillets with mushrooms and pickle. Cut the onions into thinly sliced pieces. Spread the onions over the fish fillets. Combine the stock, soy sauce, vinegar, sea salt, and stevia. Sprinkle the mixture over the fish fillets. Place the fish fillets into your air fryer and cook at 350°Fahrenheit for 10-minutes. Serve warm.

Nutrition: Calories: 278, Total Fat: 9.2g, Carbs: 7.4g, Protein: 33.2g

Chapter 12.   Vegetables & Side Dishes

Easy Veggie Fried Balls

Preparation Time: 30 minutes

Servings: 3

Nutrition:364 Calories; 13.7g Fat; 48.3g Carbs; 14g Protein; 5.3g Sugars

Ingredients

1/2 pound sweet potatoes, grated

1 cup carrots

1 cup corn

2 garlic cloves, minced

1 shallot, chopped

Sea salt and ground black pepper, to taste

2 tablespoons fresh parsley, chopped

1 egg, well beaten

1/2 cup purpose flour

1/2 cup Romano cheese, grated

1/2 cup dried bread flakes

1 tablespoon olive oil

Directions

Mix the veggies, spices, egg, flour, and Romano cheese until everything is well incorporated.

Take 1 tablespoon of the veggie mixture and roll into a ball. Roll the balls onto the dried bread flakes. Brush the veggie balls with olive oil on all sides.

Cook in the preheated Air Fryer at 360 degrees F for 15 minutes or until thoroughly cooked and crispy.

Repeat the process until you run out of ingredients. Bon appétit!

Fried Peppers with Sriracha Mayo

Preparation Time: 20 minutes

Servings: 2

Nutrition:346 Calories; 34.1g Fat; 9.5g Carbs; 2.3g Protein; 4.9g Sugars

Ingredients

4 bell peppers, seeded and sliced (1-inch pieces

1 onion, sliced (1-inch pieces

1 tablespoon olive oil

1/2 teaspoon dried rosemary

1/2 teaspoon dried basil

Kosher salt, to taste

1/4 teaspoon ground black pepper

1/3 cup mayonnaise

1/3 teaspoon Sriracha

Directions

Toss the bell peppers and onions with the olive oil, rosemary, basil, salt, and black pepper.

Place the peppers and onions on an even layer in the cooking basket. Cook at 400 degrees F for 12 to 14 minutes.

Meanwhile, make the sauce by whisking the mayonnaise and Sriracha. Serve immediately.

Classic Fried Pickles

Preparation Time: 20 minutes

Servings: 2

Nutrition:342 Calories; 28.5g Fat; 12.5g Carbs; 9.1g Protein; 4.9g Sugars

Ingredients

1 egg, whisked

2 tablespoons buttermilk

1/2 cup fresh breadcrumbs

1/4 cup Romano cheese, grated

1/2 teaspoon onion powder

1/2 teaspoon garlic powder

1 ½ cups dill pickle chips, pressed dry with kitchen towels

Mayo Sauce:

1/4 cup mayonnaise

1/2 tablespoon mustard

1/2 teaspoon molasses

1 tablespoon ketchup

1/4 teaspoon ground black pepper

Directions

In a shallow bowl, whisk the egg with buttermilk.

In another bowl, mix the breadcrumbs, cheese, onion powder, and garlic powder.

Dredge the pickle chips in the egg mixture, then, in the breadcrumb/cheese mixture.

Cook in the preheated Air Fryer at 400 degrees F for 5 minutes; shake the basket and cook for 5 minutes more.

Meanwhile, mix all the sauce ingredients until well combined. Serve the fried pickles with the mayo sauce for dipping.

Fried Green Beans with Pecorino Romano

Preparation Time: 15 minutes

Servings: 3

Nutrition:340 Calories; 9.7g Fat; 50.9g Carbs; 12.8g Protein; 4.7g Sugars

Ingredients

2 tablespoons buttermilk

1 egg

4 tablespoons cornmeal

4 tablespoons tortilla chips, crushed

4 tablespoons Pecorino Romano cheese, finely grated

Coarse salt and crushed black pepper, to taste

1 teaspoon smoked paprika

12 ounces green beans, trimmed

Directions

In a shallow bowl, whisk together the buttermilk and egg.

In a separate bowl, combine the cornmeal, tortilla chips, Pecorino Romano cheese, salt, black pepper, and paprika.

Dip the green beans in the egg mixture, then, in the cornmeal/cheese mixture. Place the green beans in the lightly greased cooking basket.

Cook in the preheated Air Fryer at 390 degrees F for 4 minutes. Shake the basket and cook for a further 3 minutes.

Taste, adjust the seasonings, and serve with the dipping sauce if desired. Bon appétit!

Spicy Roasted Potatoes

Preparation Time: 15 minutes

Servings: 2

Nutrition:299 Calories; 13.6g Fat; 40.9g Carbs; 4.8g Protein; 1.4g Sugars

Ingredients

4 potatoes, peeled and cut into wedges

2 tablespoons olive oil

Sea salt and ground black pepper, to taste

1 teaspoon cayenne pepper

1/2 teaspoon ancho chili powder

Directions

Toss all ingredients in a mixing bowl until the potatoes are well covered.

Transfer them to the Air Fryer basket and cook at 400 degrees F for 6 minutes; shake the basket and cook for a further 6 minutes.

Serve warm with your favorite sauce for dipping. Bon appétit!

Spicy Glazed Carrots

Preparation Time: 20 minutes

Servings: 3

Nutrition:162 Calories; 9.3g Fat; 20.1g Carbs; 1.4g Protein; 12.8g Sugars

Ingredients

1 pound carrots, cut into matchsticks

2 tablespoons peanut oil

1 tablespoon agave syrup

1 jalapeño, seeded and minced

1/4 teaspoon dill

1/2 teaspoon basil

Salt and white pepper to taste

Directions

Start by preheating your Air Fryer to 380 degrees F.

Toss all ingredients together and place them in the Air Fryer basket.

Cook for 15 minutes, shaking the basket halfway through the cooking time. Transfer to a serving platter and enjoy!

Easy Sweet Potato Bake

Preparation Time: 35 minutes

Servings: 3

Nutrition:409 Calories; 26.1g Fat; 38.3g Carbs; 7.2g Protein; 10.9g Sugars

Ingredients

1 stick butter, melted

1 pound sweet potatoes, mashed

2 tablespoons honey

2 eggs, beaten

1/3 cup coconut milk

1/4 cup flour

1/2 cup fresh breadcrumbs

Directions

Start by preheating your Air Fryer to 325 degrees F.

Spritz a casserole dish with cooking oil.

In a mixing bowl, combine all ingredients, except for the breadcrumbs and 1 tablespoon of butter. Spoon the mixture into the prepared casserole dish.

Top with the breadcrumbs and brush the top with the remaining 1 tablespoon of butter. Bake in the preheated Air Fryer for 30 minutes. Bon appétit!

Avocado Fries with Roasted Garlic Mayonnaise

Preparation Time: 50 minutes

Servings: 4

Nutrition:351 Calories; 27.7g Fat; 21.5g Carbs; 6.4g Protein; 1.1g Sugars

Ingredients

1/2 head garlic (6-7 cloves

3/4 cup all-purpose flour

Sea salt and ground black pepper, to taste

2 eggs

1 cup tortilla chips, crushed

3 avocados, cut into wedges

Sauce:

1/2 cup mayonnaise

1 teaspoon lemon juice

1 teaspoon mustard

Directions

Place the garlic on a piece of aluminum foil and spritz with cooking spray. Wrap the garlic in the foil.

Cook in the preheated Air Fryer at 400 degrees for 12 minutes. Check the garlic, open the top of the foil and continue to cook for 10 minutes more.

Let it cool for 10 to 15 minutes; remove the cloves by squeezing them out of the skins; mash the garlic and reserve.

In a shallow bowl, combine the flour, salt, and black pepper. In another shallow dish, whisk the eggs until frothy.

Place the crushed tortilla chips in a third shallow dish. Dredge the avocado wedges in the flour mixture, shaking off the excess. Then, dip in the egg mixture; lastly, dredge in crushed tortilla chips.

Spritz the avocado wedges with cooking oil on all sides.

Cook in the preheated Air Fryer at 395 degrees F approximately 8 minutes, turning them over halfway through the cooking time.

Meanwhile, combine the sauce ingredients with the smashed roasted garlic. To serve, divide the avocado fries between plates and top with the sauce. Enjoy!

Roasted Broccoli with Sesame Seeds

Preparation Time: 15 minutes

Servings: 2

Nutrition:267 Calories; 19.5g Fat; 20.2g Carbs; 8.9g Protein; 5.2g Sugars

Ingredients

1 pound broccoli florets

2 tablespoons sesame oil

1/2 teaspoon shallot powder

1/2 teaspoon porcini powder

1 teaspoon garlic powder

Sea salt and ground black pepper, to taste

1/2 teaspoon cumin powder

1/4 teaspoon paprika

2 tablespoons sesame seeds

Directions

Start by preheating the Air Fryer to 400 degrees F.

Blanch the broccoli in salted boiling water until al dente, about 3 to 4 minutes. Drain well and transfer to the lightly greased Air Fryer basket.

Add the sesame oil, shallot powder, porcini powder, garlic powder, salt, black pepper, cumin powder, paprika, and sesame seeds.

Cook for 6 minutes, tossing halfway through the cooking time. Bon appétit!

Corn on the Cob with Herb Butter

Preparation Time: 15 minutes

Servings: 2

Nutrition:239 Calories; 13.3g Fat; 30.2g Carbs; 5.4g Protein; 5.8g Sugars

Ingredients

2 ears fresh corn, shucked and cut into halves

2 tablespoons butter, room temperature

1 teaspoon granulated garlic

1/2 teaspoon fresh ginger, grated

Sea salt and ground black pepper, to taste

1 tablespoon fresh rosemary, chopped

1 tablespoon fresh basil, chopped

2 tablespoons fresh chives, roughly chopped

Directions

Spritz the corn with cooking spray. Cook at 395 degrees F for 6 minutes, turning them over halfway through the cooking time.

In the meantime, mix the butter with the granulated garlic, ginger, salt, black pepper, rosemary, and basil.

Spread the butter mixture all over the corn on the cob. Cook in the preheated Air Fryer an additional 2 minutes. Bon appétit!

Rainbow Vegetable Fritters

Preparation Time: 20 minutes

Servings: 2

Nutrition:215 Calories; 8.4g Fat; 31.6g Carbs; 6g Protein; 4.1g Sugars

Ingredients

1 zucchini, grated and squeezed

1 cup corn kernels

1/2 cup canned green peas

4 tablespoons all-purpose flour

2 tablespoons fresh shallots, minced

1 teaspoon fresh garlic, minced

1 tablespoon peanut oil

Sea salt and ground black pepper, to taste

1 teaspoon cayenne pepper

Directions

In a mixing bowl, thoroughly combine all ingredients until everything is well incorporated.

Shape the mixture into patties. Spritz the Air Fryer basket with cooking spray.

Cook in the preheated Air Fryer at 365 degrees F for 6 minutes. Turn them over and cook for a further 6 minutes

Serve immediately and enjoy!

Mediterranean Vegetable Skewers

Preparation Time: 30 minutes

Servings: 4

Nutrition:138 Calories; 10.2g Fat; 10.2g Carbs; 2.2g Protein; 6.6g Sugars

Ingredients

2 medium-sized zucchini, cut into 1-inch pieces

2 red bell peppers, cut into 1-inch pieces

1 green bell pepper, cut into 1-inch pieces

1 red onion, cut into 1-inch pieces

2 tablespoons olive oil

Sea salt, to taste

1/2 teaspoon black pepper, preferably freshly cracked

1/2 teaspoon red pepper flakes

Directions

Soak the wooden skewers in water for 15 minutes.

Thread the vegetables on skewers; drizzle olive oil all over the vegetable skewers; sprinkle with spices.

Cook in the preheated Air Fryer at 400 degrees F for 13 minutes. Serve warm and enjoy!

Roasted Veggies with Yogurt-Tahini Sauce

Preparation Time: 20 minutes

Servings: 4

Nutrition:254 Calories; 17.2g Fat; 19.6g Carbs; 11.1g Protein; 8.1g Sugars

Ingredients

1 pound Brussels sprouts

1 pound button mushrooms

2 tablespoons olive oil

1/2 teaspoon white pepper

1/2 teaspoon dried dill weed

1/2 teaspoon cayenne pepper

1/2 teaspoon celery seeds

1/2 teaspoon mustard seeds

Salt, to taste

Yogurt Tahini Sauce:

1 cup plain yogurt

2 heaping tablespoons tahini paste

1 tablespoon lemon juice

1 tablespoon extra-virgin olive oil

1/2 teaspoon Aleppo pepper, minced

Directions

Toss the Brussels sprouts and mushrooms with olive oil and spices. Preheat your Air Fryer to 380 degrees F.

Add the Brussels sprouts to the cooking basket and cook for 10 minutes.

Add the mushrooms, turn the temperature to 390 degrees and cook for 6 minutes more.

While the vegetables are cooking, make the sauce by whisking all ingredients. Serve the warm vegetables with the sauce on the side. Bon appétit!

Swiss Cheese & Vegetable Casserole

Preparation Time: 50 minutes

Servings: 4

Nutrition:328 Calories; 16.5g Fat; 33.1g Carbs; 13.1g Protein; 7.6g Sugars

Ingredients

1 pound potatoes, peeled and sliced (1/4-inch thick

2 tablespoons olive oil

1/2 teaspoon red pepper flakes, crushed

1/2 teaspoon freshly ground black pepper

Salt, to taste

3 bell peppers, thinly sliced

1 serrano pepper, thinly sliced

2 medium-sized tomatoes, sliced

1 leek, thinly sliced

2 garlic cloves, minced

1 cup Swiss cheese, shredded

Directions

Start by preheating your Air Fryer to 350 degrees F. Spritz a casserole dish with cooking oil.

Place the potatoes in the casserole dish in an even layer; drizzle 1 tablespoon of olive oil over the top. Then, add the red pepper, black pepper, and salt.

Add 2 bell peppers and 1/2 of the leeks. Add the tomatoes and the remaining 1 tablespoon of olive oil.

Add the remaining peppers, leeks, and minced garlic. Top with the cheese.

Cover the casserole with foil and bake for 32 minutes. Remove the foil and increase the temperature to 400 degrees F; bake an additional 16 minutes. Bon appétit!

Easy Sweet Potato Hash Browns

Preparation Time: 50 minutes

Servings: 2

Nutrition:381 Calories; 16.7g Fat; 44.8g Carbs; 14.3g Protein; 3.9g Sugars

Ingredients

1 pound sweet potatoes, peeled and grated

2 eggs, whisked

1/4 cup scallions, chopped

1 teaspoon fresh garlic, minced

Sea salt and ground black pepper, to taste

1/4 teaspoon ground allspice

1/2 teaspoon cinnamon

1 tablespoon peanut oil

Directions

Allow the sweet potatoes to soak for 25 minutes in cold water. Drain the water; dry the sweet potatoes with a kitchen towel.

Add the remaining ingredients and stir to combine well.

Cook in the preheated Air Fryer at 395 degrees F for 20 minutes. Shake the basket once or twice. Serve with ketchup.

American-Style Brussel Sprout Salad

Preparation Time: 35 minutes

Servings: 4

Nutrition:319 Calories; 18.5g Fat; 27g Carbs; 14.7g Protein; 14.6g Sugars

Ingredients

1 pound Brussels sprouts

1 apple, cored and diced

1/2 cup mozzarella cheese, crumbled

1/2 cup pomegranate seeds

1 small-sized red onion, chopped

4 eggs, hardboiled and sliced

Dressing:

1/4 cup olive oil

2 tablespoons champagne vinegar

1 teaspoon Dijon mustard

1 teaspoon honey

Sea salt and ground black pepper, to taste

Directions

Start by preheating your Air Fryer to 380 degrees F.

Add the Brussels sprouts to the cooking basket. Spritz with cooking spray and cook for 15 minutes. Let it cool to room temperature about 15 minutes.

Toss the Brussels sprouts with the apple, cheese, pomegranate seeds, and red onion.

Mix all ingredients for the dressing and toss to combine well. Serve topped with the hard-boiled eggs. Bon appétit!

The Best Cauliflower Tater Tots

Preparation Time: 25 minutes

Servings: 4

Nutrition:267 Calories; 19.2g Fat; 9.6g Carbs; 14.9g Protein; 2.9g Sugars

Ingredients

1 pound cauliflower florets

2 eggs

1 tablespoon olive oil

2 tablespoons scallions, chopped

1 garlic clove, minced

1 cup Colby cheese, shredded

1/2 cup breadcrumbs

Sea salt and ground black pepper, to taste

1/4 teaspoon dried dill weed

1 teaspoon paprika

Directions

Blanch the cauliflower in salted boiling water about 3 to 4 minutes until al dente. Drain well and pulse in a food processor.

Add the remaining ingredients; mix to combine well. Shape the cauliflower mixture into bite-sized tots.

Spritz the Air Fryer basket with cooking spray.

Cook in the preheated Air Fryer at 375 degrees F for 16 minutes, shaking halfway through the cooking time. Serve with your favorite sauce for dipping. Bon appétit!

Skinny Pumpkin Chips

Preparation Time: 20 minutes

Servings: 2

Nutrition:118 Calories; 7g Fat; 14.7g Carbs; 2.2g Protein; 6.2g Sugars

Ingredients

1 pound pumpkin, cut into sticks

1 tablespoon coconut oil

1/2 teaspoon rosemary

1/2 teaspoon basil

Salt and ground black pepper, to taste

Directions

Start by preheating the Air Fryer to 395 degrees F. Brush the pumpkin sticks with coconut oil; add the spices and toss to combine.

Cook for 13 minutes, shaking the basket halfway through the cooking time.

Serve with mayonnaise. Bon appétit!

Cheese Stuffed Roasted Peppers

Preparation Time: 20 minutes

Servings: 2

Nutrition:367 Calories; 21.8g Fat; 21.9g Carbs; 21.5g Protein; 14.1g Sugars

Ingredients

2 red bell peppers, tops and seeds removed

2 yellow bell peppers, tops and seeds removed

Salt and pepper, to taste

1 cup cream cheese

4 tablespoons mayonnaise

2 pickles, chopped

Directions

Arrange the peppers in the lightly greased cooking basket. Cook in the preheated Air Fryer at 400 degrees F for 15 minutes, turning them over halfway through the cooking time.

Season with salt and pepper.

Then, in a mixing bowl, combine the cream cheese with the mayonnaise and chopped pickles. Stuff the pepper with the cream cheese mixture and serve. Enjoy!

Three-Cheese Stuffed Mushrooms

Preparation Time: 15 minutes

Servings: 3

Nutrition:345 Calories; 28g Fat; 11.2g Carbs; 14.4g Protein; 8.1g Sugars

Ingredients

9 large button mushrooms, stems removed

1 tablespoon olive oil

Salt and ground black pepper, to taste

1/2 teaspoon dried rosemary

6 tablespoons Swiss cheese shredded

6 tablespoons Romano cheese, shredded

6 tablespoons cream cheese

1 teaspoon soy sauce

1 teaspoon garlic, minced

3 tablespoons green onion, minced

Directions

Brush the mushroom caps with olive oil; sprinkle with salt, pepper, and rosemary.

In a mixing bowl, thoroughly combine the remaining ingredients; mix to combine well and divide the filling mixture among the mushroom caps.

Cook in the preheated Air Fryer at 390 degrees F for 7 minutes.

Let the mushrooms cool slightly before serving. Bon appétit!

Sweet Potato Chips with Greek Yogurt Dip

Preparation Time: 20 minutes

Servings: 2

Nutrition:378 Calories; 13.9g Fat; 55.2g Carbs; 9.4g Protein; 12.6g Sugars

Ingredients

4 sweet potatoes, sliced

2 tablespoons olive oil

Coarse sea salt and freshly ground black pepper, to taste

1 teaspoon paprika

Dipping Sauce:

1/2 cup Greek-style yogurt

1 clove garlic, minced

1 tablespoon fresh chives, chopped

Directions

Soak the sweet potato slices in icy cold water for 20 to 30 minutes. Drain the sweet potatoes and pat them dry with kitchen towels.

Toss the sweet potato slices with olive oil, salt, black pepper, and paprika.

Place in the lightly greased cooking basket. Cook in the preheated Air Fryer at 360 degrees F for 14 minutes.

Meanwhile, make the sauce by whisking the remaining ingredients. Serve the sweet potato chips with the sauce for dipping and enjoy!

Classic Onion Rings

Preparation Time: 30 minutes

Servings: 2

Nutrition:440 Calories; 12.7g Fat; 60g Carbs; 19.2g Protein; 5.6g Sugars

Ingredients

1 medium-sized onion, slice into rings

1 cup all-purpose flour

1 teaspoon baking powder

Coarse sea salt and ground black pepper, to your liking

1/2 cup yogurt

2 eggs, beaten

3/4 cup bread crumbs

1 teaspoon onion powder

1 teaspoon garlic powder

1/2 teaspoon celery seeds

Directions

Place the onion rings in the bowl with cold water; let them soak approximately 20 minutes; drain the onion rings and pat dry using a pepper towel.

In a shallow bowl, mix the flour, baking powder, salt, and black pepper. Add the yogurt and eggs and mix well to combine.

In another shallow bowl, mix the bread crumbs, onion powder, garlic powder, and celery seeds. Dip the onion rings in the flour/egg mixture; then, dredge in the breadcrumb mixture.

Spritz the Air Fryer basket with cooking spray; arrange the breaded onion rings in the basket.

Cook in the preheated Air Fryer at 400 degrees F for 4 to 5 minutes, turning them over halfway through the cooking time. Bon appétit!

Greek-Style Roasted Tomatoes with Feta

Preparation Time: 20 minutes

Servings: 2

Nutrition:148 Calories; 9.4g Fat; 9.4g Carbs; 7.8g Protein; 6.6g Sugars

Ingredients

3 medium-sized tomatoes, cut into four slices, pat dry

1 teaspoon dried basil

1 teaspoon dried oregano

1/4 teaspoon red pepper flakes, crushed

1/2 teaspoon sea salt

3 slices Feta cheese

Directions

Spritz the tomatoes with cooking oil and transfer them to the Air Fryer basket. Sprinkle with seasonings.

Cook at 350 degrees F approximately 8 minutes turning them over halfway through the cooking time.

Top with the cheese and cook an additional 4 minutes. Bon appétit!

Sweet Corn Fritters with Avocado

Preparation Time: 20 minutes

Servings: 3

Nutrition:383 Calories; 21.3g Fat; 42.8g Carbs; 12.7g Protein; 9.2g Sugars

Ingredients

2 cups sweet corn kernels

1 small-sized onion, chopped

1 garlic clove, minced

2 eggs, whisked

1 teaspoon baking powder

2 tablespoons fresh cilantro, chopped

Sea salt and ground black pepper, to taste

1 avocado, peeled, pitted and diced

2 tablespoons sweet chili sauce

Directions

In a mixing bowl, thoroughly combine the corn, onion, garlic, eggs, baking powder, cilantro, salt, and black pepper.

Shape the corn mixture into 6 patties and transfer them to the lightly greased Air Fryer basket.

Cook in the preheated Air Fry at 370 degrees for 8 minutes; turn them over and cook for 7 minutes longer.

Serve the fritters with the avocado and chili sauce.

Cauliflower and Goat Cheese Croquettes

Preparation Time: 30 minutes

Servings: 2

Nutrition:297 Calories; 21.7g Fat; 11.7g Carbs; 15.3g Protein; 2.6g Sugars

Ingredients

1/2 pound cauliflower florets

2 garlic cloves, minced

1 cup goat cheese, shredded

Sea salt and ground black pepper, to taste

1/2 teaspoon shallot powder

1/4 teaspoon cumin powder

1 cup sour cream

1 teaspoon Dijon mustard

Directions

Place the cauliflower florets in a saucepan of water; bring to the boil; reduce the heat and cook for 10 minutes or until tender.

Mash the cauliflower using your blender; add the garlic, cheese, and spices; mix to combine well.

Form the cauliflower mixture into croquettes shapes.

Cook in the preheated Air Fryer at 375 degrees F for 16 minutes, shaking halfway through the cooking time. Serve with the sour cream and mustard. Bon appétit!

Greek-Style Vegetable Bake

Preparation Time: 35 minutes

Servings: 4

Nutrition:296 Calories; 22.9g Fat; 16.1g Carbs; 9.3g Protein; 9.9g Sugars

Ingredients

1 eggplant, peeled and sliced

2 bell peppers, seeded and sliced

1 red onion, sliced

1 teaspoon fresh garlic, minced

4 tablespoons olive oil

1 teaspoon mustard

1 teaspoon dried oregano

1 teaspoon smoked paprika

Salt and ground black pepper, to taste

1 tomato, sliced

6 ounces halloumi cheese, sliced lengthways

Directions

Start by preheating your Air Fryer to 370 degrees F. Spritz a baking pan with nonstick cooking spray.

Place the eggplant, peppers, onion, and garlic on the bottom of the baking pan. Add the olive oil, mustard, and spices. Transfer to the cooking basket and cook for 14 minutes.

Top with the tomatoes and cheese; increase the temperature to 390 degrees F and cook for 5 minutes more until bubbling. Let it sit on a cooling rack for 10 minutes before serving.

Bon appétit!

Japanese Tempura Bowl

Preparation Time: 20 minutes

Servings: 3

Nutrition:446 Calories; 14.7g Fat; 63.5g Carbs; 14.6g Protein; 3.8g Sugars

Ingredients

1 cup all-purpose flour

Kosher salt and ground black pepper, to taste

1/2 teaspoon paprika

2 eggs

3 tablespoons soda water

1 cup panko crumbs

2 tablespoons olive oil

1 cup green beans

1 onion, cut into rings

1 zucchini, cut into slices

2 tablespoons soy sauce

1 tablespoon mirin

1 teaspoon dashi granules

Directions

In a shallow bowl, mix the flour, salt, black pepper, and paprika. In a separate bowl, whisk the eggs and soda water. In a third shallow bowl, combine the panko crumbs with olive oil.

Dip the vegetables in flour mixture, then in the egg mixture; lastly, roll over the panko mixture to coat evenly.

Cook in the preheated Air Fryer at 400 degrees F for 10 minutes, shaking the basket halfway through the cooking time. Work in batches until the vegetables are crispy and golden brown.

Then, make the sauce by whisking the soy sauce, mirin, and dashi granules. Bon appétit!

Balsamic Root Vegetables

Preparation Time: 25 minutes

Servings: 3

Nutrition:405 Calories; 9.7g Fat; 74.7g Carbs; 7.7g Protein; 15.2g Sugars

Ingredients

2 potatoes, cut into 1 1/2-inch pieces

2 carrots, cut into 1 1/2-inch pieces

2 parsnips, cut into 1 1/2-inch pieces

1 onion, cut into 1 1/2-inch pieces

Pink Himalayan salt and ground black pepper, to taste

1/4 teaspoon smoked paprika

1 teaspoon garlic powder

1/2 teaspoon dried thyme

1/2 teaspoon dried marjoram

2 tablespoons olive oil

2 tablespoons balsamic vinegar

Directions

Toss all ingredients in a large mixing dish.

Roast in the preheated Air Fryer at 400 degrees F for 10 minutes. Shake the basket and cook for 7 minutes more.

Serve with some extra fresh herbs if desired. Bon appétit!

Winter Vegetable Braise

Preparation Time: 25 minutes

Servings: 2

Nutrition:358 Calories; 12.3g Fat; 55.7g Carbs; 7.7g Protein; 7.4g Sugars

Ingredients

4 potatoes, peeled and cut into 1-inch pieces

1 celery root, peeled and cut into 1-inch pieces

1 cup winter squash

2 tablespoons unsalted butter, melted

1/2 cup chicken broth

1/4 cup tomato sauce

1 teaspoon parsley

1 teaspoon rosemary

1 teaspoon thyme

Directions

Start by preheating your Air Fryer to 370 degrees F. Add all ingredients in a lightly greased casserole dish. Stir to combine well.

Bake in the preheated Air Fryer for 10 minutes. Gently stir the vegetables with a large spoon and increase temperature to 400 degrees F; cook for 10 minutes more.

Serve in individual bowls with a few drizzles of lemon juice. Bon appétit!

Family Vegetable Gratin

Preparation Time: 35 minutes

Servings: 4

Nutrition:373 Calories; 26.1g Fat; 17.7g Carbs; 18.7g Protein; 7.7g Sugars

Ingredients

1 pound Chinese cabbage, roughly chopped

2 bell peppers, seeded and sliced

1 jalapeno pepper, seeded and sliced

1 onion, thickly sliced

2 garlic cloves, sliced

1/2 stick butter

4 tablespoons all-purpose flour

1 cup milk

1 cup cream cheese

Sea salt and freshly ground black pepper, to taste

1/2 teaspoon cayenne pepper

1 cup Monterey Jack cheese, shredded

Directions

Heat a pan of salted water and bring to a boil. Boil the Chinese cabbage for 2 to 3 minutes. Transfer the Chinese cabbage to cold water to stop the cooking process.

Place the Chinese cabbage in a lightly greased casserole dish. Add the peppers, onion, and garlic.

Next, melt the butter in a saucepan over a moderate heat. Gradually add the flour and cook for 2 minutes to form a paste.

Slowly pour in the milk, stirring continuously until a thick sauce forms. Add the cream cheese. Season with the salt, black pepper, and cayenne pepper. Add the mixture to the casserole dish.

Top with the shredded Monterey Jack cheese and bake in the preheated Air Fryer at 390 degrees F for 25 minutes. Serve hot.

Roasted Beet Salad

Preparation Time: 20 minutes + chilling time

Servings: 2

Nutrition:149 Calories; 6.5g Fat; 20.6g Carbs; 3.5g Protein; 13.9g Sugars

Ingredients

2 medium-sized beets, peeled and cut into wedges

2 tablespoons extra virgin olive oil

1 tablespoon balsamic vinegar

1 teaspoon yellow mustard

1 garlic clove, minced

1/4 teaspoon cumin powder

Coarse sea salt and ground black pepper, to taste

1 tablespoon fresh parsley leaves, roughly chopped

Directions

Place the beets in a single layer in the lightly greased cooking basket.

Cook at 370 degrees F for 13 minutes, shaking the basket halfway through the cooking time.

Let it cool to room temperature; toss the beets with the remaining ingredients. Serve well chilled. Enjoy!

Spicy Ricotta Stuffed Mushrooms

Preparation Time: 35 minutes

Servings: 4

Nutrition:214 Calories; 5.6g Fat; 30.4g Carbs; 12.3g Protein; 5g Sugars

Ingredients

1/2 pound small white mushrooms

Sea salt and ground black pepper, to taste

2 tablespoons Ricotta cheese

1/2 teaspoon ancho chili powder

1 teaspoon paprika

4 tablespoons all-purpose flour

1 egg

1/2 cup fresh breadcrumbs

Directions

Remove the stems from the mushroom caps and chop them; mix the chopped mushrooms steams with the salt, black pepper, cheese, chili powder, and paprika.

Stuff the mushroom caps with the cheese filling.

Place the flour in a shallow bowl, and beat the egg in another bowl. Place the breadcrumbs in a third shallow bowl.

Dip the mushrooms in the flour, then, dip in the egg mixture; finally, dredge in the breadcrumbs and press to adhere. Spritz the stuffed mushrooms with cooking spray.

Cook in the preheated Air Fryer at 360 degrees F for 18 minutes. Bon appétit!

Baked Cholula Cauliflower

Preparation Time: 20 minutes

Servings: 4

Nutrition:153 Calories; 7.3g Fat; 19.3g Carbs; 4.1g Protein; 2.9g Sugars

Ingredients

1/2 cup all-purpose flour

1/2 cup water

Salt, to taste

1/2 teaspoon ground black pepper

1/2 teaspoon shallot powder

1/2 teaspoon garlic powder

1/2 teaspoon cayenne pepper

2 tablespoons olive oil

1 pound cauliflower, broken into small florets

1/4 cup Cholula sauce

Directions

Start by preheating your Air Fryer to 400 degrees F. Lightly grease a baking pan with cooking spray.

In a mixing bowl, combine the flour, water, spices, and olive oil. Coat the cauliflower with the prepared batter; arrange the cauliflower on the baking pan.

Then, bake in the preheated Air Fryer for 8 minutes or until golden brown.

Brush the Cholula sauce all over the cauliflower florets and bake an additional 4 to 5 minutes. Bon appétit!

Fall Vegetables with Spiced Yogurt

Preparation Time: 25 minutes

Servings: 2

Nutrition:319 Calories; 14.1g Fat; 46g Carbs; 6.4g Protein; 20.1g Sugars

Ingredients

1 pound celeriac, cut into 1 1/2-inch pieces

2 carrots, cut into 1 1/2-inch pieces

2 red onions, cut into 1 1/2-inch pieces

1 tablespoon sesame oil

1/2 teaspoon ground black pepper, to taste

1/2 teaspoon sea salt

Spiced Yogurt:

1/4 cup Greek yogurt

1 tablespoon mayonnaise

1 tablespoon honey

1/2 teaspoon mustard seeds

1/2 teaspoon chili powder

Directions

Place the vegetables in a single layer in the lightly greased cooking basket. Drizzle the sesame oil over vegetables.

Sprinkle with black pepper and sea salt.

Cook at 390 degrees F for 20 minutes, shaking the basket halfway through the cooking time.

Meanwhile, make the sauce by whisking all ingredients. Spoon the sauce over the roasted vegetables. Bon appétit!

Sweet-and-Sour Mixed Veggies

Preparation Time: 25 minutes

Servings: 4

Nutrition:153 Calories; 7.1g Fat; 21.6g Carbs; 3.6g Protein; 14.2g Sugars

Ingredients

1/2 pound asparagus, cut into 1 1/2-inch pieces

1/2 pound broccoli, cut into 1 1/2-inch pieces

1/2 pound carrots, cut into 1 1/2-inch pieces

2 tablespoons peanut oil

Some salt and white pepper, to taste

1/2 cup water

4 tablespoons raisins

2 tablespoon honey

2 tablespoons apple cider vinegar

Directions

Place the vegetables in a single layer in the lightly greased cooking basket. Drizzle the peanut oil over the vegetables.

Sprinkle with salt and white pepper.

Cook at 380 degrees F for 15 minutes, shaking the basket halfway through the cooking time.

Add 1/2 cup of water to a saucepan; bring to a rapid boil and add the raisins, honey, and vinegar. Cook for 5 to 7 minutes or until the sauce has reduced by half.

Spoon the sauce over the warm vegetables and serve immediately. Bon appétit!

Roasted Corn Salad

Preparation Time: 15 minutes + chilling time

Servings: 3

Nutrition:205 Calories; 9.5g Fat; 27g Carbs; 7.5g Protein; 7.9g Sugars

Ingredients

2 ears of corn, husked

3 tablespoons sour cream

1/4 cup plain yogurt

1 garlic clove, minced

1 jalapeño pepper, seeded and minced

1 tablespoon fresh lemon juice

Pink salt and white pepper, to your liking

1 shallot, chopped

2 bell peppers, seeded and thinly sliced

2 tablespoons fresh parsley, chopped

1/4 cup Queso Fresco, crumbled

Directions

Start by preheating the Air Fryer to 390 degrees F. Spritz the Air Fryer grill pan with cooking spray.

Place the corn on the grill pan and cook for 10 minutes, turning over halfway through the cooking time. Set aside.

Once the corn has cooled to the touch, use a sharp knife to cut off the kernels into a salad bowl.

While the corn is resting, whisk the sour cream, yogurt, garlic, jalapeño pepper, fresh lemon juice, salt, and white pepper.

Add the shallot, pepper, and parsley to the salad bowl and toss to combine well. Toss with the sauce and serve topped with cheese. Enjoy!

Rainbow Vegetable and Parmesan Croquettes

Preparation Time: 40 minutes

Servings: 4

Nutrition:377 Calories; 19.1g Fat; 40.2g Carbs; 12.1g Protein; 3.9g Sugars

Ingredients

1 pound potatoes, peeled

4 tablespoons milk

2 tablespoons butter

Salt and black pepper, to taste

1/2 teaspoon cayenne pepper

1/2 cup mushrooms, chopped

1/4 cup broccoli, chopped

1 carrot, grated

1 clove garlic, minced

3 tablespoons scallions, minced

2 tablespoons olive oil

1/2 cup all-purpose flour

2 eggs

1/2 cup panko bread crumbs

1/2 cup parmesan cheese, grated

Directions

In a large saucepan, boil the potatoes for 17 to 20 minutes. Drain the potatoes and mash with the milk, butter, salt, black pepper, and cayenne pepper.

Add the mushrooms, broccoli, carrots, garlic, scallions, and olive oil; stir to combine well. Shape the mixture into patties.

In a shallow bowl, place the flour; beat the eggs in another bowl; in a third bowl, combine the breadcrumbs with the parmesan cheese.

Dip each patty into the flour, followed by the eggs, and then the breadcrumb mixture; press to adhere.

Cook in the preheated Air Fryer at 375 degrees F for 16 minutes, shaking halfway through the cooking time. Bon appétit!

Crispy Wax Beans with Almonds and Blue Cheese

Preparation Time: 15 minutes

Servings: 3

Nutrition:242 Calories; 16.9g Fat; 16.3g Carbs; 6.8g Protein; 3.5g Sugars

Ingredients

1 pound wax beans, cleaned

2 tablespoons peanut oil

4 tablespoons seasoned breadcrumbs

Sea salt and ground black pepper, to taste

1/2 teaspoon red pepper flakes, crushed

2 tablespoons almonds, sliced

1/3 cup blue cheese, crumbled

Directions

Toss the wax beans with the peanut oil, breadcrumbs, salt, black pepper, and red pepper.

Place the wax beans in the lightly greased cooking basket.

Cook in the preheated Air Fryer at 400 degrees F for 5 minutes. Shake the basket once or twice.

Add the almonds and cook for 3 minutes more or until lightly toasted. Serve topped with blue cheese and enjoy!

Indian Malai Kofta

Preparation Time: 40 minutes

Servings: 4

Nutrition:338 Calories; 13.1g Fat; 46.8g Carbs; 10.9g Protein; 9.2g Sugars

Ingredients

Veggie Balls:

1 pound potatoes, peeled and diced

1/2 pound cauliflower, broken into small florets

2 tablespoons olive oil

2 cloves garlic, minced

1 tablespoon Garam masala

1 cup chickpea flour

Himalayan pink salt and ground black pepper, to taste

Sauce:

1 tablespoon sesame oil

1/2 teaspoon cumin seeds

2 cloves garlic, roughly chopped

1 onion, chopped

1 Kashmiri chili pepper, seeded and minced

1 (1-inch piece ginger, chopped

1 teaspoon paprika

1 teaspoon turmeric powder

2 ripe tomatoes, pureed

1/2 cup vegetable broth

1/4 full fat coconut milk

Directions

Start by preheating your Air Fryer to 400 degrees F. Place the potato and cauliflower in a lightly greased cooking basket.

Cook for 15 minutes, shaking the basket halfway through the cooking time. Mash the cauliflower and potatoes in a mixing bowl.

Add the remaining ingredients for the veggie balls and stir to combine well. Shape the vegetable mixture into small balls and arrange them in the cooking basket.

Cook in the preheated Air Fryer at 360 degrees F for 15 minutes or until thoroughly cooked and crispy. Repeat the process until you run out of ingredients.

Heat the sesame oil in a saucepan over medium heat and add the cumin seeds. Once the cumin seeds turn brown, add the garlic, onions, chili pepper, and ginger. Sauté for 2 to 3 minutes.

Add the paprika, turmeric powder, tomatoes, and broth; let it simmer, covered, for 4 to 5 minutes, stirring occasionally.

Add the coconut milk. Heat off; add the veggie balls and gently stir to combine. Bon appétit!

Carrot and Oat Balls

Preparation Time: 25 minutes

Servings: 3

Nutrition:215 Calories; 4.7g Fat; 37.2g Carbs; 7.5g Protein; 5.6g Sugars

Ingredients

4 carrots, grated

1 cup rolled oats, ground

1 tablespoon butter, room temperature

1 tablespoon chia seeds

1/2 cup scallions, chopped

2 cloves garlic, minced

2 tablespoons tomato ketchup

1 teaspoon cayenne pepper

1/2 teaspoon sea salt

1/4 teaspoon ground black pepper

1/2 teaspoon ancho chili powder

1/4 cup fresh bread crumbs

Directions

Start by preheating your Air Fryer to 380 degrees F.

In a bowl, mix all ingredients until everything is well incorporated. Shape the batter into bite-sized balls.

Cook the balls for 15 minutes, shaking the basket halfway through the cooking time. Bon appétit!

Sweet Potato and Chickpea Tacos

Preparation Time: 15 minutes

Servings: 4

Nutrition:427 Calories; 26.6g Fat; 34.4g Carbs; 15.3g Protein; 4.5g Sugars

Ingredients

2 cups sweet potato puree

2 tablespoons butter, melted

14 ounces canned chickpeas, rinsed

1 cup Colby cheese, shredded

1 teaspoon garlic powder

1 teaspoon onion powder

Salt and freshly cracked black pepper, to taste

8 corn tortillas

1/4 cup Pico de gallo

2 tablespoons fresh coriander, chopped

Directions

Mix the sweet potatoes with the butter, chickpeas, cheese, garlic powder, onion powder, salt, black pepper.

Divide the sweet potato mixture between the tortillas. Bake in the preheated Air Fryer at 390 degrees F for 7 minutes.

Garnish with Pico de gallo and coriander. Bon appétit!

Kid-Friendly Veggie Tots

Preparation Time: 20 minutes

Servings: 4

Nutrition:222 Calories; 14.2g Fat; 18.3g Carbs; 5.7g Protein; 3.5g Sugars

Ingredients

1 zucchini, grated

1 parsnip, grated

1 carrot, grated

1 onion, chopped

1 garlic clove, minced

2 tablespoons ground flax seeds

2 eggs, whisked

1/2 cup tortilla chips, crushed

1/4 cup pork rinds

Sea salt and ground black pepper, to taste

Directions

Start by preheating your Air Fryer to 400 degrees F.

Then, in a mixing bowl, thoroughly combine all ingredients until everything is well combined. Form the mixture into tot shapes and place in the lightly greased cooking basket.

Bake for 9 to 12 minutes, flipping halfway through, until golden brown around the edges. Bon appétit!

Quick Shrimp and Vegetable Bake

Preparation Time: 25 minutes

Servings: 4

Nutrition:269 Calories; 8.8g Fat; 21.7g Carbs; 28.2g Protein; 12g Sugars

Ingredients

1 pound shrimp cleaned and deveined

1 cup broccoli, cut into florets

1 cup cauliflower, cut into florets

1 carrot, sliced

2 bell pepper, sliced

1 shallot, sliced

2 tablespoons sesame oil

1 cup tomato paste

Directions

Start by preheating your Air Fryer to 360 degrees F. Spritz the baking pan with cooking spray.

Now, arrange the shrimp and vegetables in the baking pan. Then, drizzle the sesame oil over the vegetables. Pour the tomato paste over the vegetables.

Cook for 10 minutes in the preheated Air Fryer. Stir with a large spoon and cook for a further 12 minutes. Serve warm.

Roasted Brussels Sprout Salad

Preparation Time: 35 minutes + chilling time

Servings: 2

Nutrition:316 Calories; 16.6g Fat; 33.2g Carbs; 13.8g Protein; 17.7g Sugars

Ingredients

1/2 pound Brussels sprouts

1 tablespoon olive oil

Coarse sea salt and ground black pepper, to taste

2 ounces baby arugula

1 shallot, thinly sliced

2 ounces pancetta, chopped

Lemon Vinaigrette:

2 tablespoons extra virgin olive oil

2 tablespoons fresh lemon juice

1 tablespoon honey

1 teaspoon Dijon mustard

Directions

Start by preheating your Air Fryer to 380 degrees F.

Add the Brussels sprouts to the cooking basket. Brush with olive oil and cook for 15 minutes. Let it cool to room temperature about 15 minutes.

Toss the Brussels sprouts with the salt, black pepper, baby arugula, and shallot.

Mix all ingredients for the dressing. Then, dress your salad, garnish with pancetta, and serve well chilled. Bon appétit!

Winter Bliss Bowl

Preparation Time: 45 minutes

Servings: 3

Nutrition:387 Calories; 25.3g Fat; 38.5g Carbs; 6g Protein; 5.8g Sugars

Ingredients

1 cup pearled barley

1 (1-pound head cauliflower, broken into small florets

Coarse sea salt and ground black pepper, to taste

2 tablespoons champagne vinegar

4 tablespoons mayonnaise

1 teaspoon yellow mustard

4 tablespoons olive oil, divided

10 ounces ounce canned sweet corn, drained

2 tablespoons cilantro leaves, chopped

Directions

Cook the barley in a saucepan with salted water. Bring to a boil and cook approximately 28 minutes. Drain and reserve.

Start by preheating the Air Fryer to 400 degrees F.

Place the cauliflower florets in the lightly greased Air Fryer basket. Season with salt and black pepper; cook for 12 minutes, tossing halfway through the cooking time.

Toss with the reserved barley. Add the champagne vinegar, mayonnaise, mustard, olive oil, and corn. Garnish with fresh cilantro. Bon appétit!

Tater Tot Vegetable Casserole

Preparation Time: 40 minutes

Servings: 6

Nutrition:493 Calories; 26.1g Fat; 49.6g Carbs; 17.1g Protein; 5.7g Sugars

Ingredients

1 tablespoon olive oil

1 shallot, sliced

2 cloves garlic, minced

1 red bell pepper, seeded and sliced

1 yellow bell pepper, seeded and sliced

1 ½ cups kale

1 (28-ounce bag frozen tater tots

6 eggs

1 cup milk

Sea salt and ground black pepper, to your liking

1 cup Swiss cheese, shredded

4 tablespoons seasoned breadcrumbs

Directions

Heat the olive oil in a saucepan over medium-high heat. Sauté the shallot, garlic, and peppers for 2 to 3 minutes. Add the kale and cook until wilted.

Arrange the tater tots evenly over the bottom of a lightly greased casserole dish. Spread the sautéed mixture over the top.

In a mixing bowl, thoroughly combine the eggs, milk, salt, pepper, and shredded cheese. Pour the mixture into the casserole dish.

Lastly, top with the seasoned breadcrumbs. Bake at 330 degrees F for 30 minutes or until top is golden brown. Bon appétit!

Fried Asparagus with Goat Cheese

Preparation Time: 15 minutes

Servings: 3

Nutrition:132 Calories; 11.2g Fat; 2.2g Carbs; 6.5g Protein; 1g Sugars

Ingredients

1 bunch of asparagus, trimmed

1 tablespoon olive oil

1/2 teaspoon kosher salt

1/4 teaspoon cracked black pepper, to taste

1/2 teaspoon dried dill weed

1/2 cup goat cheese, crumbled

Directions

Place the asparagus spears in the lightly greased cooking basket. Toss the asparagus with the olive oil, salt, black pepper, and dill.

Cook in the preheated Air Fryer at 400 degrees F for 9 minutes.

Serve garnished with goat cheese. Bon appétit!

Cheesy Crusted Baked Eggplant

Preparation Time: 45 minutes

Servings: 3

Nutrition:233 Calories; 7.6g Fat; 29.3g Carbs; 12.9g Protein; 7.4g Sugars

Ingredients

1 pound eggplant, sliced

1 tablespoon sea salt

1/4 cup Romano cheese, preferably freshly grated

1/3 cup breadcrumbs

Sea salt and cracked black pepper, to taste

1 egg, whisked

4 tablespoons cornmeal

1/4 cup mozzarella cheese, grated

2 tablespoons fresh Italian parsley, roughly chopped

Directions

Toss the eggplant with 1 tablespoon of salt and let it stand for 30 minutes. Drain and rinse.

Mix the cheese, breadcrumbs, salt, and black pepper in a bowl. Then, add the whisked egg and cornmeal.

Dip the eggplant slices in the batter and press to coat on all sides. Transfer to the lightly greased Air Fryer basket.

Cook at 370 degrees F for 7 to 9 minutes. Turn each slice over and top with the mozzarella. Cook an additional 2 minutes or until the cheese melts.

Serve garnished with fresh Italian parsley. Bon appétit!

Asian Fennel and Noodle Salad

Preparation Time: 20 minutes + chilling time

Servings: 3

Nutrition:248 Calories; 13.2g Fat; 29.9g Carbs; 3.7g Protein; 12.7g Sugars

Ingredients

1 fennel bulb, quartered

Salt and white pepper, to taste

1 clove garlic, finely chopped

1 green onion, thinly sliced

2 cups Chinese cabbage, shredded

2 tablespoons rice wine vinegar

1 tablespoon honey

2 tablespoons sesame oil

1 teaspoon ginger, freshly grated

1 tablespoon soy sauce

1 cup chow mein noodles, for serving

Directions

Start by preheating your Air Fryer to 370 degrees F.

Now, cook the fennel bulb in the lightly greased cooking basket for 15 minutes, shaking the basket once or twice.

Let it cool completely and toss with the remaining ingredients. Serve well chilled.

Italian Peperonata Classica

Preparation Time: 25 minutes

Servings: 4

Nutrition:389 Calories; 18.4g Fat; 49.1g Carbs; 9.3g Protein; 19.8g Sugars

Ingredients

2 tablespoons olive oil

4 bell peppers, seeded and sliced

1 serrano pepper, seeded and sliced

1/2 cup onion, peeled and sliced

2 garlic cloves, crushed

2 tomatoes, pureed

2 tablespoons tomato ketchup

Sea salt and black pepper

1 teaspoon cayenne pepper

4 fresh basil leaves

10 Sicilian olives green, pitted and sliced

2 Ciabatta rolls

Directions

Brush the sides and bottom of the cooking basket with 1 tablespoon of olive oil. Add the peppers, onions, and garlic to the cooking basket. Cook for 5 minutes or until tender.

Add the tomatoes, ketchup, salt, black pepper, and cayenne pepper; add the remaining tablespoon of olive oil and cook in the preheated Air Fryer at 380 degrees F for 15 minutes, stirring occasionally.

Divide between individual bowls and garnish with basil leaves and olives. Serve with the Ciabatta rolls. Bon appétit!

Cheesy Scalloped Potatoes

Preparation Time: 45 minutes

Servings: 4

Nutrition:470 Calories; 22g Fat; 50.1g Carbs; 18.6g Protein; 8.7g Sugars

Ingredients

4 medium potatoes

2 tablespoons butter

2 tablespoons all-purpose flour

1 cup milk

1 cup half-and-half

Sea salt and red pepper flakes, to taste

1/2 teaspoon shallot powder

1/2 teaspoon garlic powder

1 ½ cups Colby cheese, shredded

Directions

Bring a large pot of water to a boil. Cook the whole potatoes for about 20 minutes. Drain the potatoes and let sit until cool enough to handle.

Peel your potatoes and slice into 1/8-inch rounds. Melt the butter in a pan over a moderate flame; add the flour and cook for 1 minute. Slowly and gradually, whisk in the milk; cook until the sauce has thickened.

Add the half-and-half, salt, red pepper, shallot powder, and garlic powder.

Place 1/2 of the potatoes overlapping in a single layer in the lightly greased casserole dish. Spoon 1/2 of the cheese sauce on top of the potatoes. Repeat the layers.

Top with the shredded cheese. Bake in the preheated Air Fryer at 325 degrees F for 20 minutes. Serve warm.

Twice-Baked Potatoes with Pancetta

Preparation Time: 30 minutes

Servings: 5

Nutrition:401 Calories; 7.7g Fat; 69.9g Carbs; 15.2g Protein; 3.8g Sugars

Ingredients

2 teaspoons canola oil

5 large russet potatoes, peeled

Sea salt and ground black pepper, to taste

5 slices pancetta, chopped

5 tablespoons Swiss cheese, shredded

Directions

Start by preheating your Air Fryer to 360 degrees F.

Drizzle the canola oil all over the potatoes. Place the potatoes in the Air Fryer basket and cook approximately 20 minutes, shaking the basket periodically.

Lightly crush the potatoes to split and season them with salt and ground black pepper. Add the pancetta and cheese.

Place in the preheated Air Fryer and bake an additional 5 minutes or until cheese has melted. Bon appétit!

Charred Asparagus and Cherry Tomato Salad

Preparation Time: 10 minutes + chilling time

Servings: 4

Nutrition:289 Calories; 16.7g Fat; 30.1g Carbs; 8.9g Protein; 19.9g Sugars

Ingredients

1/4 cup olive oil

1 pound asparagus, trimmed

1 pound cherry tomatoes

1/4 cup balsamic vinegar

2 garlic cloves, minced

2 scallion stalks, chopped

1/2 teaspoon oregano

Coarse sea salt and ground black pepper, to your liking

2 hard-boiled eggs, sliced

Directions

Start by preheating your Air Fryer to 400 degrees F. Brush the cooking basket with 1 tablespoon of olive oil.

Add the asparagus and cherry tomatoes to the cooking basket. Drizzle 1 tablespoon of olive oil all over your veggies.

Cook for 5 minutes, shaking the basket halfway through the cooking time. Let it cool slightly.

Toss with the remaining olive oil, balsamic vinegar, garlic, scallions, oregano, salt, and black pepper.

Afterwards, add the hard-boiled eggs on the top of your salad and serve.

Skinny Breaded Baby Portabellas

Preparation Time: 15 minutes

Servings: 4

Nutrition:260 Calories; 6.4g Fat; 39.2g Carbs; 12.1g Protein; 5.8g Sugars

Ingredients

1 ½ pounds baby portabellas

1/2 cup cornmeal

1/2 cup all-purpose flour

2 eggs

2 tablespoons milk

1 cup breadcrumbs

Sea salt and ground black pepper

1/2 teaspoon shallot powder

1 teaspoon garlic powder

1/2 teaspoon cumin powder

1/2 teaspoon cayenne pepper

Directions

Pat the mushrooms dry with a paper towel.

To begin, set up your breading station. Mix the cornmeal and all-purpose flour in a shallow dish. In a separate dish, whisk the eggs with milk.

Finally, place your breadcrumbs and seasonings in the third dish.

Start by dredging the baby portabellas in the flour mixture; then, dip them into the egg wash. Press the baby portabellas into the breadcrumbs, coating evenly.

Spritz the Air Fryer basket with cooking oil. Add the baby portabellas and cook at 400 degrees F for 6 minutes, flipping them halfway through the cooking time. Bon appétit!

Crispy Parmesan Asparagus

Preparation Time: 20 minutes

Servings: 4

Nutrition:207 Calories; 12.4g Fat; 11.7g Carbs; 12.2g Protein; 1.6g Sugars

Ingredients

2 eggs

1 teaspoon Dijon mustard

1 cup Parmesan cheese, grated

1 cup bread crumbs

Sea salt and ground black pepper, to taste

18 asparagus spears, trimmed

1/2 cup sour cream

Directions

Start by preheating your Air Fryer to 400 degrees F.

In a shallow bowl, whisk the eggs and mustard. In another shallow bowl, combine the Parmesan cheese, breadcrumbs, salt, and black pepper.

Dip the asparagus spears in the egg mixture, then in the parmesan mixture; press to adhere.

Cook for 5 minutes; work in three batches. Serve with sour cream on the side. Enjoy!

Chapter 13.   Desserts

Tasty Banana Cake

Preparation time: 40 Minutes

Servings: 4

Ingredients

1 tbsp. butter, soft

1 egg

1/3 cup brown sugar

2 tbsp. honey

1 banana

1 cup white flour

1 tbsp. baking powder

½ tbsp. cinnamon powder

Cooking spray

Instructions

Spurt cake pan with cooking spray.

Mix in butter with honey, sugar, banana, cinnamon, egg, flour and baking powder in a bowl then beat.

Empty mix in cake pan with cooking spray, put into air fryer and cook at 350°F for 30 minutes.

Allow for cooling, slice.

Serve.

Simple Cheesecake

Preparation time: 25 Minutes

Servings: 15

Ingredients

1 lb. cream cheese

½ tbsp. vanilla extract

2 eggs

4 tbsp. sugar

1 cup graham crackers

2 tbsp. butter

Instructions

Mix in butter with crackers in a bowl.

Compress crackers blend to the bottom cake pan, put into air fryer and cook at 350° F for 4 minutes.

Mix cream cheese with sugar, vanilla, egg in a bowl and beat properly.

Sprinkle filling on crackers crust and cook cheesecake in air fryer at 310° F for 15 minutes.

Keep cake in fridge for 3 hours, slice.

Serve.

Bread Pudding

Preparation time: 10 Minutes

Servings: 4

Ingredients

6 glazed doughnuts

1 cup cherries

4 egg yolks

1 and ½ cups whipping cream

½ cup raisins

¼ cup sugar

½ cup chocolate chips.

Instructions

Mix in cherries with whipping cream and egg in a bowl then turn properly.

Mix in raisins with chocolate chips, sugar and doughnuts in a bowl then stir.

Mix the 2 mixtures, pour into oiled pan then into air fryer and cook at 310° F for 1 hour.

Cool pudding before cutting.

Serve.

Bread Dough and Amaretto Dessert

Preparation time: 22 Minutes

Servings: 12

Ingredients

1 lb. bread dough

1 cup sugar

½ cup butter

1 cup heavy cream

12 oz. chocolate chips

2 tbsp. amaretto liqueur

Instructions

Turn dough, cut into 20 slices and cut each piece in halves.

Sweep dough pieces with spray sugar, butter, put into air fryer's basket and cook them at 350°F for 5 minutes. Turn them, cook for 3 minutes still. Move to a platter.

Melt the heavy cream in pan over medium heat, put chocolate chips and turn until they melt.

Put in liqueur, turn and move to a bowl.

Serve bread dippers with the sauce.

Wrapped Pears

Preparation time: 10 Minutes

Servings: 4

Ingredients

4 puff pastry sheets

14 oz. vanilla custard

2 pears

1 egg

½ tbsp. cinnamon powder

2 tbsp. sugar

Instructions

Put wisp pastry slices on flat surface, add spoonful of vanilla custard at the center of each, add pear halves and wrap.

Sweep pears with egg, cinnamon and spray sugar, put into air fryer's basket and cook at 320°F for 15 minutes.

Split parcels on plates.

Serve.

Air Fried Bananas

Preparation time: 10 Minutes

Servings: 4

Ingredients

3 tbsp. butter

2 eggs

8 bananas

½ cup corn flour

3 tbsp. cinnamon sugar

1 cup panko

Instructions

Warm up pan with the butter over medium heat, put panko, turn and cook for 4 minutes then move to a bowl.

Spin each in flour, panko, egg blend, assemble them in air fryer's basket, grime with cinnamon sugar and cook at 280° F for 10 minutes.

Serve immediately.

Cocoa Cake

Preparation time: 10 Minutes

Servings: 6

Ingredients

3.5 oz. butter

3 eggs

3 oz. sugar

1 tbsp. cocoa powder

3 oz. flour

½ tbsp. lemon juice

Instructions

Mix in 1 tablespoon butter with cocoa powder in a bowl and beat.

Mix in the rest of the butter with eggs, flour, sugar and lemon juice in another bowl, blend properly and move half into a cake pan

Put half of the cocoa blend, spread, add the rest of the butter layer and crest with remaining cocoa.

Put into air fryer and cook at 360° F for 17 minutes.

Allow to cool before slicing.

Serve.

Apple Bread

Preparation time: 10 Minutes

Servings: 6

Ingredients

3 cups apples

1 cup sugar

1 tbsp. vanilla

2 eggs

1 tbsp. apple pie spice

2 cups white flour

1 tbsp. baking powder

1 stick butter

1 cup water

Instructions

Mix in egg with 1 butter stick, sugar, apple pie spice and turn using mixer.

Put apples and turn properly.

Mix baking powder with flour in another bowl and turn.

Blend the 2 mixtures, turn and move it to spring form pan.

Get spring form pan into air fryer and cook at 320°F for 40 minutes

Slice.

Serve.

Banana Bread

Preparation time: 10 Minutes

Servings: 6

Ingredients

¾ cup sugar

1/3 cup butter

1 tbsp. vanilla extract

1 egg

2 bananas

1 tbsp. baking powder

1 and ½ cups flour

½ tbsp. baking soda

1/3 cup milk

1 and ½ tbsp. cream of tartar

Cooking spray

Instructions

Mix in milk with cream of tartar, vanilla, egg, sugar, bananas and butter in a bowl and turn whole.

Mix in flour with baking soda and baking powder.

Blend the 2 mixtures, turn properly, move into oiled pan with cooking spray, put into air fryer and cook at 320°F for 40 minutes.

Remove bread, allow to cool, slice.

Serve.

Mini Lava Cakes

Preparation time: 10 Minutes

Servings: 3

Ingredients

1 egg

4 tbsp. sugar

2 tbsp. olive oil

4 tbsp. milk

4 tbsp. flour

1 tbsp. cocoa powder

½ tbsp. baking powder

½ tbsp. orange zest

Instructions

Mix in egg with sugar, flour, salt, oil, milk, orange zest, baking powder and cocoa powder, turn properly. Move it to oiled ramekins.

Put ramekins in air fryer and cook at 320°F for 20 minutes.

Serve warm.

Crispy Apples

Preparation time: 10 Minutes

Servings: 4

Ingredients

2 tbsp. cinnamon powder

5 apples

½ tbsp. nutmeg powder

1 tbsp. maple syrup

½ cup water

4 tbsp. butter

¼ cup flour

¾ cup oats

¼ cup brown sugar

Instructions

Get the apples in a pan, put in nutmeg, maple syrup, cinnamon and water.

Mix in butter with flour, sugar, salt and oat, turn, put spoonful of blend over apples, get into air fryer and cook at 350°F for 10 minutes.

Serve while warm.

Ginger Cheesecake

Preparation time: 2 hours and 30 Minutes

Servings: 6

Ingredients

2 tbsp. butter

½ cup ginger cookies

16 oz. cream cheese

2 eggs

½ cup sugar

1 tbsp. rum

½ tbsp. vanilla extract

½ tbsp. nutmeg

Instructions

Spread pan with the butter and sprinkle cookie crumbs on the bottom.

Whisk cream cheese with rum, vanilla, nutmeg and eggs, beat properly and sprinkle the cookie crumbs.

Put in air fryer and cook at 340° F for 20 minutes.

Allow cheese cake to cool in fridge for 2 hours before slicing.

Serve.

Cocoa Cookies

Preparation time: 10 Minutes

Servings: 12

Ingredients

6 oz. coconut oil

6 eggs

3 oz. cocoa powder

2 tbsp. vanilla

½ tbsp. baking powder

4 oz. cream cheese

5 tbsp. sugar

Instructions

Mix in eggs with coconut oil, baking powder, cocoa powder, cream cheese, vanilla in a blender and sway and turn using a mixer.

Get it into a lined baking dish and into the fryer at 320°F and bake for 14 minutes.

Split cookie sheet into rectangles.

Serve.

Special Brownies

Preparation time: 10 Minutes

Servings: 4

Ingredients

1 egg

1/3 cup cocoa powder

1/3 cup sugar

7 tbsp. butter

½ tbsp. vanilla extract

¼ cup white flour

¼ cup walnuts

½ tbsp. baking powder

1 tbsp. peanut butter

Instructions

Warm pan with 6 tablespoons butter and the sugar over medium heat, turn, cook for 5 minutes, move to a bowl, put salt, egg, cocoa powder, vanilla extract, walnuts, baking powder and flour, turn mix properly and into a pan.

Mix peanut butter with one tablespoon butter in a bowl, heat in microwave for some seconds, turn properly and sprinkle brownies blend over.

Put in air fryer and bake at 320° F and bake for 17 minutes.

Allow brownies to cool, cut.

Serve.

Blueberry Scones

Preparation time: 20 Minutes

Servings: 10

Ingredients

1 cup white flour

1 cup blueberries

2 eggs

½ cup heavy cream

½ cup butter

5 tbsp. sugar

2 tbsp. vanilla extract

2 tbsp. baking powder

Instructions

Mix in flour, baking powder, salt and blueberries in a bowl and turn.

Mix heavy cream with vanilla extract, sugar, butter and eggs and turn properly.

Blend the 2 mixtures, squeeze till dough is ready, obtain 10 triangles from mix, put on baking sheet into air fryer and cook them at 320°F for 10 minutes.

Serve cold.

Chocolate Cookies

Preparation time: 10 Minutes

Servings: 12

Ingredients

1 tbsp. vanilla extract

½ cup butter

1 egg

4 tbsp. sugar

2 cups flour

½ cup unsweetened chocolate chips

Instructions

Warm pan with butter over medium heat, turn and cook for 1 minute.

Mix in egg with sugar and vanilla extract in a bowl and turn properly.

Put flour, melted butter and half of the chocolate chips and turn.

Move to a pan, sprinkle the remaining chocolate chips over, put in the fryer at 330° F and bake for 25 minutes.

Serve slices when cold.

Tasty Orange Cake

Preparation time: 42 Minutes

Servings: 12

Ingredients

6 eggs

1 orange

1 tbsp. vanilla extract

1 tbsp. baking powder

9 oz. flour

2 oz. sugar + 2 tbsp.

2 tbsp. orange zest

4 oz. cream cheese

4 oz. yogurt

Instructions

hump orange in a food processor properly.

Put 2 tablespoons sugar, flour, vanilla extract, baking powder and throb properly.

Move mix into 2 spring form pans, put in fryer and cook at 330°F for 16 minutes.

Mix in cream cheese with yogurt and orange zest and the rest of the sugar in a bowl and turn properly.

Put one cake layer on a plate, half of the cream cheese blend, then the other cake layer and the remaining cream cheese blend.

Properly rub, slice.

Serve.

Macaroons

Preparation time: 10 Minutes

Servings: 20

Ingredients

2 tbsp. sugar

4 egg whites

2 cup coconut

1 tbsp. vanilla extract

Instructions

Mix in egg whites with stevia in a bowl and whisk using mixer.

Put coconut and vanilla extract, beat again, get small balls out of mix, put in air fryer and cook at 340°F for 8 minutes.

Serve cold.

Lime Cheesecake

Preparation time: 4 hours and 14 Minutes

Servings: 10

Ingredients

2 tbsp. butter

2 tbsp. sugar

4 oz. flour

¼ cup coconut

For the filling:

1 lb. cream cheese

Zest from 1 lime

Juice form 1 lime

2 cups hot water

2 sachets lime jelly

Instructions

Mix coconut with flour, sugar and butter in a bowl, turn properly and compress mix to bottom of pan.

Get hot water in a bowl, put jelly sachets and turn till it melts.

Get cream cheese in a bowl, put lime juice, zest and jelly and beat properly.

Get mix on crust, rub, put in air fryer and cook at 300° F for 4 minutes.

Cool in fridge for 4 hours

Serve.

Easy Granola

Preparation time: 45 Minutes

Servings: 4

Ingredients

1 cup coconut

½ cup almonds

½ cup pecans

2 tbsp. sugar

½ cup pumpkin seeds

½ cup sunflower seeds

2 tbsp. sunflower oil

1 tbsp. nutmeg

1 tbsp. apple pie spice mix

Instructions

Mix pecans and almonds with pumpkin seeds, sunflower seeds, coconut, nutmeg and apple pie spice mix in a bowl and turn properly.

Warm pan with oil over medium heat, add sugar and turn properly.

Spread on coconut mix and nuts, then turn properly.

Pour mix on a lined baking sheet, put in air fryer and cook at 300° F and bake for 25 minutes.

Allow granola to cool, slice.

Serve.

Strawberry Cobbler

Preparation time: 35 Minutes

Servings: 6

Ingredients

¾ cup sugar

6 cups strawberries

1/8 tsp. baking powder

1 tbsp. lemon juice

½ cup flour

A pinch of baking soda

½ cup water

3 and ½ tbsp. olive oil

Cooking spray

Instructions

Mix in strawberries with half of sugar, put lemon juice, spray some flour in a bowl, beat and turn into baking dish and oil with cooking spray.

Mix in flour with baking powder, the rest of the sugar, and soda and turn properly.

Put the olive oil and blend with your hands.

Get ½ cup water and sprinkle over strawberries.

Put in fryer at 355°F and roast for 25 minutes.

Allow cobbler to cool, slice.

Serve.

Plum Cake

Preparation time: 1 hour and 56 Minutes

Servings: 8

Ingredients

7 oz. flour

1 pack dried yeast

1 oz. butter

1 egg

5 tbsp. sugar

3 oz. milk

1 and ¾ lbs. plums

Zest from 1 lemon

1 oz. almond flakes

Instructions

Mix in yeast with butter,3 tablespoons sugar, and flour in a bowl, then turn properly.

Put in egg and milk and beat for 4 minutes till dough is made.

Assemble the dough in a spring form pan oiled with some butter, keep for 1 hour covered.

Assemble plumps over the butter, spray the remaining sugar, put in air fryer at 350°F, bake for 36 minutes, let cool, spread lemon zest and almond flakes over, slice.

Serve.

Lentils and Dates Brownies

Preparation time: 25 Minutes

Servings: 8

Ingredients

28 oz. canned lentils

12 dates

1 tbsp. honey

1 banana

½ tbsp. baking soda

4 tbsp. almond butter

2 tbsp. cocoa powder

Instructions

Mix lentils with cocoa, banana, butter, honey and baking soda in a food processor and beat properly.

Put dates, thump for some time, get mix in oiled pan smear well, put in the fryer at 360°F and roast for 15 minutes.

Remove brownies blend from oven, slice, assemble on a platter.

Serve.

Maple Cupcakes

Preparation time: 30 Minutes

Servings: 4

Ingredients

4 tbsp. butter

4 eggs

½ cup pure applesauce

2 tbsp. cinnamon powder

1 tbsp. vanilla extract

½ apple

4 tbsp. maple syrup

¾ cup white flour

½ tbsp. baking powder

Instructions

Warm pan with the butter over medium heat, put vanilla, apple sauce, eggs and maple syrup, stir, remove heat. Allow to cool.

Put cinnamon, flour, baking powder and apples, beat, put in a cupcake pan, get in air fryer at 350°F and roast for 20 minutes.

Allow cupcakes to cool, put on a platter.

Serve.

Rhubarb Pie

Preparation time: 1 hour 15 Minutes

Servings: 6

Ingredients

1 and ¼ cups almond flour

8 tbsp. butter

5 tbsp. cold water

1 tbsp. sugar

For the filling

3 cups rhubarb

3 tbsp. flour

1 and ½ cups sugar

2 eggs

½ tbsp. nutmeg

1 tbsp. utter

2 tbsp. low fat milk

Instructions

Mix 1 and ¼ cups flour with, 8 tablespoons butter, 1 teaspoon sugar and cold water in a bowl, turn and compress till dough is made.

Move dough to a floured working surface, make disk shape, flatten, roll in plastic, allow in fridge for 30 minutes, wrap and press on the bottom of a pie pan.

Mix in rhubarb with 1 and ½ cups sugar, 8 tablespoons butter and nutmeg, then beat.

Beat milk with egg, put rhubarb blend in another bowl, put the blend into the pie crust, get into air fryer and cook at 390°F for 45 minutes.

Serve sliced and cold.

Mandarin Pudding

Preparation time: 1 hour

Servings: 8

Ingredients

1 mandarin

Juice from 2 mandarins

2 tbsp. brown sugar

4 oz. butter

2 eggs

¾ cup sugar

¾ cup white flour

¾ cup almonds

Honey for serving

Instructions

Smear a loaf pan with butter, spray brown sugar on the bottom and assemble mandarin slices.

Mix in butter with egg, sugar, almonds, mandarin juice and flour, turn, spread mix over mandarin slices, put pan in air fryer and cook at 360°F for 40 minutes.

Place pudding on plate.

Serve with honey over.

Sponge Cake

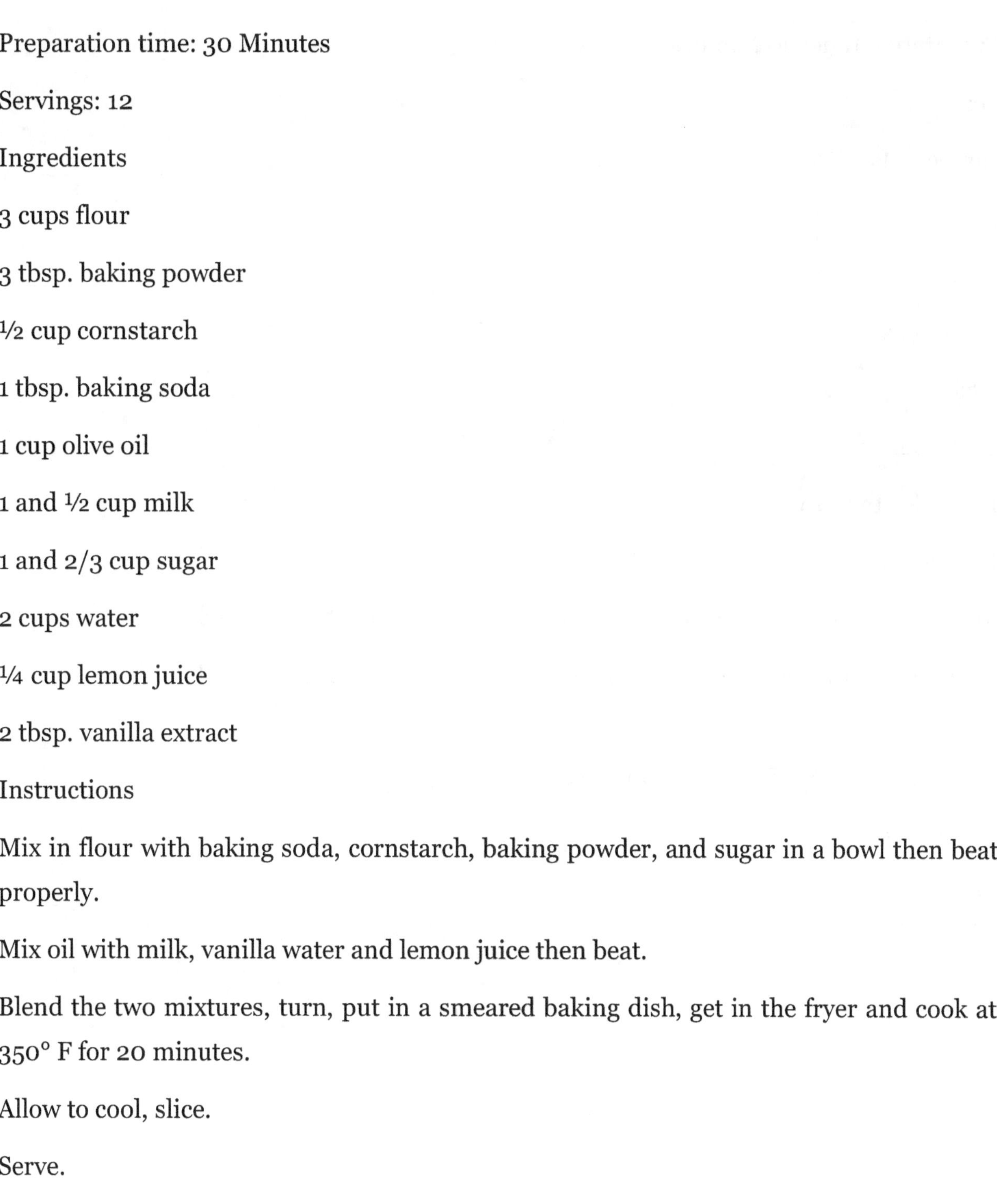

Preparation time: 30 Minutes

Servings: 12

Ingredients

3 cups flour

3 tbsp. baking powder

½ cup cornstarch

1 tbsp. baking soda

1 cup olive oil

1 and ½ cup milk

1 and 2/3 cup sugar

2 cups water

¼ cup lemon juice

2 tbsp. vanilla extract

Instructions

Mix in flour with baking soda, cornstarch, baking powder, and sugar in a bowl then beat properly.

Mix oil with milk, vanilla water and lemon juice then beat.

Blend the two mixtures, turn, put in a smeared baking dish, get in the fryer and cook at 350° F for 20 minutes.

Allow to cool, slice.

Serve.

Ricotta and Lemon Cake

Preparation time: 20 Minutes

Servings: 4

Ingredients

8 eggs

3 lbs. ricotta cheese

½ lb. sugar

Zest from 1 lemon

Zest from 1 orange

Butter for the pan

Instructions

Mix in eggs with lemon sugar, orange zest and cheese, then turn properly.

Smear pan with some batter, spray ricotta mix, get in the fryer at 39° F and roast for 30 minutes.

Lessen heat at 380°F and roast for 40 minutes still.

Remove from oven, allow to cool.

Serve.

Almond cupcake

Preparation time: 5 minutes

Cooking time: 20 minutes

Servings: 3 to 5 people

Ingredients:

3 tablespoons of butter

2 tablespoons of real maple syrup

½ cup of almond flour

1/8 teaspoon of salt

1/3 cup of chocolate chips

1 egg beaten

½ teaspoon of vanilla

Directions:

Preheat oven to 350 degrees. Place cupcake liners into the pan. Preheat to 3200F. Use silicone cupcake liners.

In a glass or stainless steel bowl, add the chocolate chips, butter and honey and heat over a double boiler for a few seconds just until the chocolate starts to melt.

Remove the bowl when the chocolate begins to melt and begin stirring until the butter, honey and chocolate are well blended.

Let cool for approximately 5 to 8 minutes. Add the remaining ingredients to the cooled melted chocolate and stir well with a wooden spoon.

Scoop the batter into the prepared cupcake pan. Bake for about 15 to 18 minutes, or until an inserted toothpick comes out clean.

If toothpick does not come out clean, continue to cook for about 3 to 4 minute intervals. Top with slivered almonds and unsweetened shredded coconut.

Sprinkle with powdered sugar and serve.

Lava Cake

Preparation time: 5 minutes

Cooking time: 10 minutes

Servings: 2 to 4 people

Ingredients:

1 egg

2 tbsp. of cocoa powder

2 tbsp. of water

2 tbsp. of non-GMO erythritol

1/8 tsp. of Stevia

1 tbsp. of golden flax meal

1 tbsp. of coconut oil, melted

½ tsp. of aluminum-free baking powder

Dash of vanilla

Pinch of Himalayan salt

Directions:

Whisk all ingredients in a two-cup glass Pyrex dish or ramekin.

Preheat air fryer at 350°F for just a minute. Place glass dish with cake mix into air fryer and bake at 350°F for about 8 to 9 minutes.

Carefully remove dish with an oven mitt. Let cool for a few minutes and then enjoy!

Chocolate cake

Preparation time: 10 minutes

Cooking time: 55 minutes

Overall time: 1 hour 5 minutes

Servings: 2 to 4 people

Ingredients:

3 large eggs

1 cup (128g of almond flour

2/3 cup (85g of sugar

1/3 cup (78ml of heavy cream

¼ cup (59ml of coconut oil melted

¼ cup (32g of unsweetened cocoa powder

1 teaspoon of baking powder

½ teaspoon of orange zest

1/8 cup (16g of chopped walnuts

1/8 cup (16g of chopped pecans

Unsalted butter at room temperature

Directions:

Butter a 7-inch round baking pan and line the bottom with parchment paper.

Place all ingredients into a large bowl. With a hand mixer on medium speed, beat until the batter is light and fluffy.

This is important for preventing the cake from being too dense. Carefully fold the nuts into the batter to keep the air in.

Pour cake batter into the pan and cover tightly with aluminum foil. Place in the air fryer basket and cook for about 45 minutes at 3250F.

Remove the foil and then cook for an additional 10 to 15 minutes, until a knife inserted in the center comes out clean.

Take pan out of air fryer and set on a cooling rack for 10 minutes. Then remove cake from the pan and let it cool for additional 20 minutes. Slice and serve.

Blueberry hand pie

Preparation time: 15 minutes

Cooking time: 12 minutes

Servings: 2 to 4 people

Ingredients:

1 cup (128g of blueberries

2.5 tablespoon of caster sugar

1 teaspoon of lemon juice

1 pinch salt

14 oz. (320g of refrigerated pie crust or shortcrust pastry roll

Water

Vanilla sugar to sprinkle on top (optional

Directions:

Mix together the blueberries, sugar, lemon juice, and salt in a medium bowl.

Roll out the piecrusts and cut out 6-8 (4-inch individual circles. Place about 1 tablespoon of the blueberry filling in the center of each circle.

Moisten edges of dough with water, and fold the dough over the filling to form a half moon shape. Using a fork, gently crimp the edges of the piecrust together.

Then cut three slits on the top of the hand pies. Spray the hand pies with cooking spray and sprinkle with vanilla sugar.

Preheat the air fryer to 3500F. Place 3-4 hand pies in single layer inside the air fryer basket. Cook for about 9 to 12 minutes, or until golden brown.

Let the pies cool for at least 10 minutes before serving.

Nutella Smores

Preparation time: 2 minutes

Cooking time:5 minutes

Overall time: 7 minutes

Servings: 2 to 4 people

Ingredients:

4 graham crackers cut in half

4 jumbo marshmallows, use 2 cut in half

Strawberries and Raspberries

4 teaspoons of Nutella

Directions:

Preheat the air fryer to 3500F. Place 4 graham cracker halves (or 4 biscuits in the air fryer basket.

Put 1 marshmallow on top of each graham cracker half. Cook for 5 minutes, till marshmallow is nice and golden.

Add the berries and the Nutella. Top each with a graham cracker half. Serve and enjoy!

Pop Tarts

Preparation time: 10 minutes

Cooking time: 7 minutes

Servings: 2 to 4 people

Ingredients:

1 refrigerated or homemade pie crust

½ cup of strawberry jam

Cooking spray, optional

½ cup of Greek yogurt, for icing, optional

Directions:

Lay out refrigerated pie crust or roll out homemade pie crust.

Using a cookie cutter, cut out two shapes for every pop tart you want to make. Spoon out about a tablespoon of a jam and spread it within 1/2 ″ of your edge.

Carefully place the other cutout on top of your jam and gently press edges together using a fork. Place pop tarts in the air fryer, careful that they are not touching.

Spray the top of the pop tarts if you want them to crisp a little more, but it's totally not necessarily.

Cook for about 7 to 10 minutes at 3700F, checking every minute after 6 minutes for desired doneness.

They are ready and delicious at that point, but if you want some healthier "icing," mix a dollop of fruit spread and a dollop of Greek yogurt and drizzle over the top!

Serve immediately and Enjoy!

Pumpkin French Toast

Preparation time: 4 minutes

Cooking time: 16 minutes

Servings: 1 to 3 people

Ingredients:

Air fryer grill pan

4 slices whole meal bread

1 small egg

3 tablespoons whole milk

120g of pumpkin

60g of pumpkin pie filling

2 teaspoons of honey

Pinch of nutmeg

Directions:

Chop up your fresh pumpkin into small cubes and place them into a mixing bowl.

Mix them with the honey and nutmeg until the pumpkin pieces are well coated. Place the pumpkin cubes into the Air fryer.

Cook for about 8 minutes at 3600F.In the same mixing bowl add the milk and the egg and mix well with a fork until the egg is well beaten.

Add to it the pumpkin pie filling and give it a good mix. Remove the pumpkin from the Air fryer and put to one side.

Soak the sliced bread in the French toast batter until it feels like it has drowned in it, remove any excess moisture and place it in the Air fryer via the grill pan.

Cook for about 4 minutes on one side at 4000F and then turn over with some tongs.

Once turned over add the pumpkin from earlier and cook for a further 4 minutes at the same temperature.

8.   Drizzle with extra pumpkin juices and a little honey and then serve.

Burgers

Preparation time: 15 minutes

Cooking time: 45 minutes

Servings: 2 to 4 people

Ingredients:

300g of mixed mince pork and beef

Onion

1 teaspoon of garlic puree

1 teaspoon of tomato puree

1 teaspoon of mustard

1 teaspoon of basil

1 teaspoon of mixed herbs

Salt & pepper

25g of cheddar cheese

4 bread buns

Salad for burger topping

Directions:

In a mixing bowl add the mince and seasoning and mix well.

Form into four medium sized burgers and place in the Air Fryer cooking tray. Cook in the Air Fryer on 200c for 25 minutes and then check on them.

Cook them for further 20 minutes on 1800C. Then add your salad, cheese and bun and serve!

Apple Fritters

Preparation time: 10 minutes

Cooking time: 15 minutes

Servings: 2 to 4 people

Ingredients:

Fritters

1 cup of self-rising flour

1 cup of plain Greek yogurt

2 teaspoon of sugar optional

1 tablespoon of cinnamon

1 large apple peeled and chopped

Glaze

1 cup of confectioner sugar

2 tablespoons of milk or more, if needed

Directions:

Mix all fritter ingredients together in a medium bowl. Knead the mixture in the bowl about 3 to 4 times.

Mix glaze ingredients together, this mixture should be on the thin side. Set it aside. Line the bottom of the air fryer with a parchment round.

Spray the parchment liberally with oil. Divide the fritter batter into 4 balls about the size of a handball. Flatten slightly and place in the fryer basket.

Spray with vegetable oil. Air fry at 3700F for about 13 to 15 minutes, turning half way through the cooking.

Spray with oil again after turning. Check for doneness with a toothpick. Drizzle or dip in the glaze then place fritters on a wire rack to cool and dry the glaze.

Serve immediately and Enjoy!

Mini banana bread

Preparation time: 5 minutes

Cooking time: 30 minutes

Servings: 2 to 4 people

Ingredients:

1 banana mashed (ripe

1 egg

3 tbsp. of brown sugar

2 tbsp. of canola oil

¼ cup of milk

¾ cup of plain flour mixed

½ tsp. of baking soda

Directions:

Line a very small baking tin or oven safe glass dish with baking paper and trim. Spray with a little oil. If using an oven, preheat to 3200F.

In a small bowl, whisk the egg into the mashed banana. Then whisk in the sugar, oil, and milk. Add the flour and baking soda and mix until just combined.

Pour the batter into the prepared tin, bake in your oven or air fryer for about 25 to 35 minutes or until a skewer poked into the bottom of the cake comes out clean.

For me it takes about 30 to 35 minutes in my air fryer and 25 minutes in an oven. Let cool for 10 minutes in the tin/dish, then transfer to a wire rack to cool.

Serve immediately and Enjoy!

Cherry Pies

Preparation time: 5 minutes

Cooking time: 10 minutes

Overall time:15 minutes

Servings: 2 to 4 people

Ingredients:

14-ounce package of refrigerated pie crusts

½ cup of cherry pie filling

Non-stick cooking spray

3 tbsp. of confectioner sugar

½ tsp. of milk

Directions:

Unroll refrigerated pie crusts. Cut out 6 pies with cookie cutter. Place 1.5 tablespoons cherry pie filling near the center of each piece of dough.

Fold pie in half. Seal edge by pressing lightly with tines of a fork. Make 3 small cuts in top of dough. Place in basket of air fryer.

Spray lightly with non-stick cooking spray. Cook in air fryer approximately 10 minutes at 3500F.

Remove when lightly browned. Allow to cool. Mix glaze ingredients thoroughly to remove lumps. Drizzle over top of cooled pies.

Serve immediately and Enjoy!

Brussels Sprouts

Preparation time: 5 minutes

Cooking time: 20 minutes

Servings: 2 to 4 people

Ingredients:

1 pound of Brussels sprouts cut in half

2 tablespoons of honey

1 ½ tablespoons of vegetable oil

1 tablespoon of gochujang

½ teaspoon of salt

Cooking Instructions

Combine honey, vegetable oil, gochujang, and salt in a bowl and stir. Set it aside about 1 tablespoon of the sauce.

Add Brussels sprouts to bowl and stir until all sprouts are fully covered. Place your Brussels sprouts in your Air Fryer, ensuring that they are not overlapping.

cook at 3600F for about 15 minutes, shaking the basket halfway through. Set aside the bowl.

Once 15 minutes cooking time is up, increase temperature to 3900F and cook for about 5 more minutes.

When sprouts are done, place in bowl and cover with reserved sauce and stir. Enjoy.

Sweet potato dessert fries

Preparation time: 5 minutes

Cooking time: 20 minutes

Servings: 2 to 4 people

Ingredients:

2 medium sweet potatoes

½ tbsp. of coconut oil.

1 tbsp. of arrowroot starch or cornstarch

2 tsp. of melted butter (for coating

¼ cup of coconut sugar or raw sugar

1 to 2 tbsp. of cinnamon

Powdered sugar for dusting (optional

Dipping Sauces

Dessert Hummus

Honey or Vanilla Greek Yogurt

Maple Frosting {vegan}

Directions:

Peel your sweet potatoes and wash them with clean water, then dry. Slice peeled sweet potatoes lengthwise, ½ inch thick.

Toss your sweet potato slices in 1/2 tablespoon of coconut oil and arrowroot starch (or cornstarch. Place in air fryer for about 18 minutes at 3700F.

Shake halfway at 8 to 9 minutes. Remove the fries from the air fryer and place in large bowl.

Drizzle 2 teaspoon of optional butter on top of fries. Then mix in cinnamon and sugar and toss fries together again.

Place on plate to serve, sprinkle with powdered sugar. Serve fries with dipping sauce of choice.

To store, keep fries wrapped in foil and in fridge. Then reheat in oven again to warm before serving. Should keep for 2-3 days.

Churro Bites

Preparation time: 5 minutes

Cooking time: 1 hour 5 minutes

Gross time: 1 hour 10 minutes

Servings: 2 to 4 people

Ingredients:

1 cup of water

8 tbsp. of (1 stick unsalted butter, cut into 8 pieces

½ cup of plus 1 tablespoon granulated sugar, divided

1 cup of all-purpose flour

1 tsp. of vanilla extract

3 large eggs

2 tsp. of ground cinnamon

4 oz. of finely chopped dark chocolate

¼ cup of sour cream or Greek yogurt

Directions:

Bring the water, butter, and 1 tablespoon of the sugar to a simmer in a small saucepan over medium-high heat.

Add the flour and quickly stir it in with a sturdy wooden spoon. Continue to cook, stirring constantly, until the flour smells toasted and the mixture is thick, about 3 minutes.

Transfer to a large bowl. Using the same wooden spoon, beat the flour mixture until cooled slightly but still warm, about 1 minute of constant stirring.

Stir in the vanilla. Stir in the eggs one at a time, making sure each egg is incorporated before adding the next.

Transfer the dough to a piping bag or gallon zip-top bag. Let the dough rest for 1 hour at room temperature.

Meanwhile, prepare the cinnamon sugar and chocolate sauce. Combine the cinnamon and remaining ½ cup sugar in large bowl.

Microwave the chocolate in a medium microwave-safe mixing bowl in 30-second intervals, stirring between each, until the chocolate is melted, 1 ½ to 2 minutes.

8.   Add the sour cream or yogurt and whisk until smooth. Cover and set aside. Preheat the air fryer for 10 minutes at 375°F.

Pipe the batter directly into the preheated air fryer, making 6 (3-inch pieces and piping them at least ½ -inch apart.

10. Air fry until golden-brown, for about 10 minutes. Immediately transfer the churros to the bowl of cinnamon sugar and toss to coat.

11. Repeat with air frying the remaining batter. Serve the churros warm with the dipping sauce.

Chapter 14.   Savory Pies.

Hassel Free Breakfast Pie

Preparation Time: 25 MIN

Servings: 4

Ingredients:

6 bacon, cooked and crumbled

1 thin pastry crust

3 green onions, sliced

4 eggs

1 tsp of black pepper

2 cups of milk

1 tbsp. of maple syrup

1 cup of cheddar cheese, shredded

1 potato, boiled, chopped

1 tsp of salt

Directions:

Preheat the air fryer to 390 degrees Fahrenheit.

Place the pastry crust into a baking pan. Make sure to cut off the extra edges.

Whisk the eggs in a mixing bowl for 2 minutes. Add in the milk and whisk again.

Add the onions, potato, bacon, cheese and mix well.

Season using salt and black pepper.

Stir and add the mixture on top of the crust.

Use an aluminum foil to cover. Use a knife to make two or three holes on top.

Bake in the preheated air fryer for about 10 minutes.

Let it cool down slightly and then serve.

Duckie Pie

Servings: 4

Preparation Time: 20 minutes

Cooking Time: 10 minutes

Ingredients:

2 cups leftover roast duck

¼ cup green onions, chopped

2 tablespoons hoisin sauce

1 cup flour

3 tablespoons butter

2 tablespoons water

1 egg

Directions:

Preheat air fryer to 300°F/150°C.

Mix together the roast duck, green onions and hoisin sauce and place into the Air Fryer Baking Pan.

Mix together the flour, butter and water and knead until a dough forms.

Roll out the dough until it is large enough to cover the Air Fryer Baking Pan.

Crimp the edges onto the rim of the Air Fryer Baking Pan.

Whisk the egg and brush the pie crust.

Place the Air Fryer Baking Pan into the Air Fryer Basket and set the timer for 10 minutes.

Serve and enjoy!

Chicken and Sausage Pie

Servings: 2

Preparation Time: 10 minutes

Cooking Time: 14 minutes

Ingredients:

¾ cup cooked chicken breast, shredded

1 beef sausage, sliced

½ cup potatoes, diced

¼ cup green peas

¼ cup carrots, diced

½ teaspoon paprika

½ teaspoon garlic powder

½ teaspoon onion powder

salt and pepper, to taste

1 pastry pie dough

1 egg

Directions:

Preheat the Air Fryer to 300°F/150°C.

Place the shredded chicken, sliced beef sausages, potatoes, green peas and carrots in the Air Fryer Baking Pan.

Season with the paprika, garlic powder, onion powder, salt and pepper.

Place the Air Fryer Baking Pan in the Air Fryer and set the timer for 4 minutes.

Remove from the Air Fryer and allow to cool.

Roll out the dough to be large enough to cover the Air Fryer Baking Pan.

Seal the edges so they rest on the rim of the Air Fryer Baking Pan.

Whisk the egg and brush the pie crust.

Return to the Air Fryer and set the timer for 10 minutes.

Serve and enjoy!

Grapes Pie

Preparation time: 10 minutes

Cooking time: 30 minutes

Servings: 8

Ingredients:

2 eggs, whisked

¾ cup sugar

½ cup heavy cream

¼ cup almond flour

1 cup grapes, halved

2 tablespoons butter, melted

1 teaspoon baking powder

Directions:

In a bowl, combine the eggs with the grapes, cream and the other ingredients, whisk and pour into a pie pan.

Put the pan in the air fryer, cook at 370 degrees F for 30 minutes, slice and serve warm.

Nutrition: calories 212, fat 15, fiber 2, carbs 6, protein 4

Turkey Pie

Preparation time: 10 minutes

Cooking time: 20 minutes

Servings: 4

Ingredients:

1 pound turkey breast, boneless, skinless and cubed

1 red onion, chopped

2 tomatoes, cubed

1 cup mushrooms, chopped

1 teaspoon balsamic vinegar

Salt and black pepper to the taste

1 teaspoon coriander, chopped

1 teaspoon onion powder

½ teaspoon garlic powder

1 tablespoon white flour

1 tablespoon almond milk

2 puff pastry sheets

2 tablespoons avocado oil

Directions:

Heat up a pan with half of the oil over medium heat, add the meat, onion, mushrooms and the other ingredients except the puff pastry, toss, cook for 5 minutes and take off the heat.

Place 1 puff pastry sheet on the bottom of your air fryer's pan, add the turkey mix, top with the other puff pastry sheet, brush with the remaining oil, place the pan in the fryer, cook at 370 degrees F for 15 minutes, slice and serve for lunch.

Nutrition: calories 172, fat 3.9, fiber 2.6, carbs 13.1, protein 21.3

Spinach Cheese Pie

Preparation Time: 30 minutes

Servings: 4

Ingredients:

1 cup frozen chopped spinach, drained

¼ cup heavy whipping cream.

1 cup shredded sharp Cheddar cheese.

¼ cup diced yellow onion

6 large eggs.

Directions:

Take a medium bowl, whisk eggs and add cream. Add remaining ingredients to bowl.

Pour into a 6-inch round baking dish. Place into the air fryer basket. Adjust the temperature to 320 Degrees F and set the timer for 20 minutes

Eggs will be firm and slightly browned when cooked. Serve immediately.

Nutrition: Calories: 288; Protein: 18.0g; Fiber: 1.3g; Fat: 20.0g; Carbs: 3.9g

Lemon Coconut Pie

Preparation Time: 45 minutes

Servings: 8

Ingredients:

4 oz. coconut, shredded

2 eggs, whisked

¼ cup coconut flour

¾ cup swerve

2 tbsp. butter; melted

1 tsp. lemon zest, grated

1 tsp. baking powder

1 tsp. vanilla extract

½ tsp. lemon extract

Cooking spray

Directions:

In a bowl, combine all the ingredients except the cooking spray and stir well.

Grease a pie pan that fits the air fryer with the cooking spray

Pour the mixture inside, put the pan in the air fryer and cook at 360°F for 35 minutes. Slice and serve warm.

Nutrition: Calories: 212; Fat: 15g; Fiber: 2g; Carbs: 6g; Protein: 4g

Chapter 15.   Meal Plan

DAY	BREAKFAST	LUNCH/DINNER	DESSERT
1.	Breakfast Zucchini & Cream Muffins	Air Fried Chicken Thighs	Crispy Apples
2.	Cheese & Egg Breakfast Sandwich	Chicken Cheese Fillet	Banana Bread
3.	Crispy Breakfast Avocado Fries	Roasted Pepper Salad	Apple Bread
4.	Oriental Omelet	Pineapple Pizza	Air Fried Bananas
5.	Vegetable Egg Pancake	Air Fryer Tortilla Pizza	Wrapped Pears
6.	Breakfast Cod Nuggets	Air Fried Pork Apple Balls	Bread Dough and Amaretto Dessert
7.	Breakfast Cheese Bread Cups	Hash Brown	Bread Pudding
8.	Air Fryer Scrambled Egg	Air fried steak	Simple Cheesecake
9.	Pumpkin Pie French Toast	Baked Potatoes	Tasty Banana Cake
10.	Asparagus Omelet	Churro Bites	Cocoa Cake
11.	Air Baked Eggs	Roasted Asian Broccoli	Sweet potato dessert fries
12.	Peanut Butter & Banana	Air-Fried Asparagus	Brussels Sprouts
13.	Meatballs and Creamy Potatoes	Coconut Shrimp	Cherry Pies

14.	Creamy and Cheesy Pancake	Chocolate Chip Oatmeal	Mini banana bread
15.	Vegetarian Omelet	Mushroom Rice	Apple Fritters
16.	Bacon and Cheese Rolls	Apple chips	Pumpkin French Toast
17.	Bagels	Chicken nuggets	Burgers
18.	Banana Flapjacks	Reuben Calzones	Special Brownies
19.	Baked Spinach and Ham Eggs	Stuffed Garlic Chicken	Plum Cake
20.	Cheese and Mushroom Frittata	Rosemary Citrus Chicken	Lentils and Dates Brownies
21.	Frittata	Air Fried Garlic Popcorn Chicken	Maple Cupcakes
22.	Breakfast Muffins	Macaroni Cheese Toast	Rhubarb Pie
23.	Cheese Omelette	Cheese Burger Patties	Mandarin Pudding
24.	Full English Breakfast	Grilled Cheese Corn	Churro Bites
25.	Roasted Baby Potatoes	Eggplant Fries	Nutella Smores
26.	Sweet Potato Fritters	Raspberry Balsamic Smoked Pork Chops	Pop Tarts
27.	Eggs & Cocotte on Toast	Eggplant fries	Blueberry hand pie
28.	Avocado & Blueberry Muffins	Air Fried Pita Bread Pizza	Lava Cake

Conclusion

When it comes to cooking and using a new kitchen appliance is learning the ins and out; the way that it cooks foods specifically. If you've read through this book and tried your hand at a variety of recipes, then you should by now know what using the air fryer entails. Consequently, it should only be too easy for you to expand your horizons and try out other dishes that aren't even in this book. Substitute meats, add flavors and spices. Don't be afraid to fail. That's where true creation comes from.

And what's more, you should be able to see how healthy you can eat using the air fryer. All of these recipes are far healthier than then would be where they cooked in a deep fryer or convection oven. Simply take a step and begin air-frying.